THE
ACUPUNCTURE
HANDBOOK

About the Author

ANGELA HICKS has been an acupuncturist since 1976. She is the co-founder and joint principal of the College of Integrated Chinese Medicine in Reading, one of the largest colleges in the UK, which is affiliated with Kingston University. She is the author of *The Principles of Chinese Medicine, The Principles of Acupuncture, Five Secrets of Health and Happiness* and co-author of *Healing Your Emotions* and *Five Element Constitutional Acupuncture*.

THE
ACUPUNCTURE
HANDBOOK

How acupuncture works and
how it can help you

ANGELA
HICKS

piatkus

PIATKUS

First published in Great Britain in 2005 by Piatkus Books
This paperback edition published in 2010 by Piatkus

A CIP catalogue record for this book
is available from the British Library.

ISBN 978-0-7499-4160-4

Typeset in Bembo by Phoenix Photosetting, Chatham, Kent
Printed and bound in Great Britain by
CPI Mackays, Chatham ME5 8TD

Papers used by Piatkus are natural, renewable and recyclable
products sourced from well-managed forests and certified
in accordance with the rules of the Forest Stewardship Council.

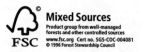

Mixed Sources
Product group from well-managed
forests and other controlled sources
www.fsc.org Cert no. SGS-COC-004081
© 1996 Forest Stewardship Council
FSC

Piatkus
An imprint of
Little, Brown Book Group
100 Victoria Embankment
London EC4Y 0DY

An Hachette UK Company
www.hachette.co.uk

www.piatkus.co.uk

Contents

Author's Note

This book is written as an informative guide to acupuncture and is not meant to be a self-help book for treatment.

I have capitalised all Chinese medicine terminology in order to differentiate it from standard English terms. For example, the Kidneys in upper case signifies the Chinese medicine term (i.e. the Kidneys and its Chinese medicine functions). The kidneys in lower case represents the kidneys as they are described in Western medicine.

My thanks to all of the people who have helped me to write this book. First, thank you to all of my own patients, the patients of Susan Tosoni, Sandy Steele, Michael Pringle, Vanessa Lampert and Jill Glover and patients of third-year students that I supervised, who talked with me about their experiences of acupuncture. The names of all patients have been changed to protect confidentiality.

Second, thanks to the practitioners who discussed information about specialised treatments: Beth Soderstrom, Soreh Levy and Carolyn MacDonald – drug dependency; Julian Scott and Celene Kershen – the treatment of children; Ann Hutchison and Geraldine Worthington – veterinary acupuncture; Diana Griffin – auricular acupuncture; Xiao Yang Zhang – guasha; David Mayor – electro-acupuncture; Jamie Hedger and Qing Zhang – facial rejuvenation; Jill Glover and Sally Blades – treatment in childbirth. Thanks also to Mark Bovey of the Acupuncture Research Resource Centre who directed me towards relevant research. Also Persis Tamboly at the BAcC who helped me with the list of professional bodies and societies, to Liong-Sen Liew for providing the Chinese characters and to Peter Eckman and Neal White for the drawings.

Third, thanks to all those who have helped me by reading this book, most notably Judith Clark for her brilliant proof-reading, Peter Mole who helped me with the 'big picture' and Jane Grossfeld who made so many helpful comments. Also thank you to Gill Bailey, Anna Crago, Jo Brooks and Helen Stanton at Piatkus for all of their help and support.

Many people have helped me to deepen my appreciation of Chinese medicine, especially J. R. Worsley. I am deeply grateful to him for his inspiration and for teaching me the importance of treating the mind and spirit as well as the body. Also thank you to others who have taught me, including doctors in China who were so helpful to me when I was learning TCM.

Thanks as well to all my friends and colleagues in the acupuncture community – it's a wonderful community that I deeply treasure.

Finally, my thanks and love to John, my husband, who is always so supportive and encouraging and to whom I dedicate this book.

Disclaimer

The contents of this book are for information only. The author recommends that you consult qualified practitioners when considering acupuncture. Do not attempt to self-treat or alter your medication without consulting your doctor. The author and publisher cannot accept any responsibility for illness or injury arising out of failure to follow these guidelines.

Introduction

I first started studying acupuncture in 1973. Now, over thirty-five years later, I run an acupuncture college in the UK and I am still as inspired and excited as I was when I began studying.

Back in 1973 acupuncture was a little-known treatment and was usually classified as a 'fringe' medicine. I was impressed to see it transform a close friend's health and, knowing I would love to help people, I trustingly decided that this would be my future career.

With no other evidence as to its beneficial effects I embarked on a three-year course of study and at the same time started a course of acupuncture treatment. I began the treatment thinking that I had no problems with my health, but that the experience of acupuncture would make me a better practitioner. It did, in fact, profoundly improve my health – something I still never forget whenever I treat other people.

When I started treatment I would not have described myself as being 'ill'. Like other 'healthy' people I never caught colds and flu and never took time off work. I felt tired and weak most of the time, but I didn't think there was anything that could be done to help that. I was also permanently anxious, but that was how I'd been for most of my life, so I accepted it. I knew I didn't always sleep well at night and I had other minor symptoms such as my terrible memory (at school I held the record for having the most belongings in lost property in one week). But poor concentration was not something I associated with poor health. More than anything else, though, I felt slightly miserable much of the time and didn't know why – like many other people, I thought this was my lot in life.

When I initially went for treatment, my practitioner asked me many questions about myself. She felt some pulses on the radial artery of my wrist and carried out other examinations to find out more about my health. She then gave me some acupuncture treatment.

My experience after the first treatment was stunning. I knew something had changed and I definitely felt much better in myself. There was something else, though, that I couldn't quite put my finger on. Finally, I realised that for a long time my life had felt totally flat. I'd carried that feeling with me for so long that I didn't even know it was there. Now for the first time in my life I felt that it was positively good to be alive!

Never again since then has that awful feeling returned, and over a period of time I felt increasingly strong physically and happier in my spirits. I look back at the younger me and know that without doubt that treatment transformed my life.

My practitioner later told me that she had diagnosed my symptoms to be coming from my Heart and Heart Protector. This didn't mean I had a heart problem in a conventional sense. I'm sure a test given by a doctor would have found nothing wrong with my heart. In Chinese medicine a Heart problem causes many different signs and symptoms – some physical and others relating to the emotions, mind or spirit.

Since that time I have given literally thousands of acupuncture treatments myself and have seen it transform the lives of many of my patients. The way lives are transformed is always individual – sometimes there is a rapid change and at other times a slow, steady but solid shift. Obviously not everyone gets completely better – but it helps large numbers of people. As you might expect, an acupuncturist considers each person to be completely unique and all treatments are tailor-made to suit the individual. Alongside a change in symptoms, patients almost always experience an increased feeling of well-being. This indicates that changes in health are arising from deep within. Later on in the book you will read other patients' accounts of the differences they experienced after treatment.

Times have really changed since those early years when I first became a practitioner. At that time acupuncture was often a last resort for patients; they only came for acupuncture when all other treatments had failed. Now it is often a patient's first choice. I have continued to benefit from treatment and, along with Qigong (Chinese exercise) and following a fairly balanced lifestyle regime, I have used it to further improve my health and to deal with any difficulties life has thrown at me. I have had other patients do the same. One of my patients, who is now 88, has been coming for treatment, and keeping herself healthy, for over 30 years. She is remarkably youthful for her age and she swears that acupuncture has contributed to keeping her from ageing.

Some time after I had finished my acupuncture studies, I started to teach. I have now been teaching both undergraduate and postgraduate students for over 30 years. In 1993 I co-founded an acupuncture college and since then I have spent most of my time running the college and teaching. The students learn about all aspects of the theory of Chinese medicine as well as being thoroughly trained in Western medicine. The course leads to a BSc honours degree in acupuncture.

When I look back, I feel proud to see how what initially seemed to be a rather strange therapy is now becoming almost a part of mainstream treatment. I also gain great satisfaction from watching students who start with a keen desire to help people blossoming into extremely competent professionals. Over their three years of study they too will have discovered how to use this wonderful treatment to transform the lives of their own patients.

I hope that by reading this book you too will 'catch' something of the magic of acupuncture. In it I will describe:

- How acupuncture can benefit your overall health and what illnesses it can treat.
- The fascinating theory of Chinese medicine and how it can be used to treat your body, mind, emotions and spirit.
- The answers to many of your frequently asked questions about treatment, such as, 'Will it hurt?' 'How are needles sterilised?' 'How long does a treatment take?' 'How do I find a practitioner?'
- How the constitutional imbalance you were born with will enable you to gain deeper insight into yourself.
- Common diagnoses and treatments for many illnesses as well as some important self-help information that you can use in your daily life.
- How acupuncture can be used to treat children and animals and can be used in childbirth, to help people who are drug dependent and is even being used for facial rejuvenation.

This book is for anyone who has an interest in acupuncture. You may be considering trying treatment yourself. You may already be having treatment and want to find out more. You may be thinking that treatment might help a friend or relative. You may even be considering studying acupuncture. Alternatively, you may just want to find out more about the theory of Chinese medicine because it is such an interesting subject.

After all of these years I still feel privileged to be teaching and using this amazing method of treatment. I hope that as you read the book just a little of this excitement is transmitted to you.

1

Introducing Acupuncture

An overview of acupuncture

Did you know as many people in the world use Chinese
Medicine as use Western medicine and for many of them it is
their first port of call when they are ill? Knowing this you may
not be surprised that acupuncture is one of the fastest growing
complementary therapies in the West.

In surveys in the UK into the use of complementary medicine it is consistently cited as one of the most commonly used
treatments. Approximately 7 per cent of the adult population in
the UK have received acupuncture and it is estimated that at
least 2 million treatments per year are carried out by private
practitioners and 1 million on the NHS.[1] But why the popularity? The key is that acupuncture works and very effectively
treats a wide range of conditions. When people receive benefit
from acupuncture they tell their friends, family and work colleagues and the word spreads.

Research carried out on 495 patients at the teaching clinic of
the College of Integrated Chinese Medicine indicates the success of the treatment. The study found that of those who had
acupuncture, a stunning 90.7 per cent said that they had expe-

rienced improvement from treatment. Of these, 56.4 percent had a major improvement or a full recovery.[2] Similar studies elsewhere concur with these results including a study of 291 acupuncture patients[3] and a study of patients with chronic pain[4]. These results, from a wide range of patients with chronic illness, indicate high levels of patient satisfaction. I will discuss more of these findings in the next chapter.

What is acupuncture?

Acupuncture is one part of the spectrum of treatments of Chinese medicine which also includes herbs, massage (*tui na*), exercise and diet. It is one of the most ancient systems of treatment known to mankind. The origins of Chinese medicine date back to at least 2,000 years ago when the first Chinese texts were written. The fact that it still survives to this day gives credence to its efficacy.

The word 'acupuncture' is derived from Latin roots. The Latin word acus means a needle and acupuncture means 'to puncture with a needle'. If you've had acupuncture you'll know that practitioners carry out treatment by inserting a few fine needles into points on your body. These points are located and linked on 'channels' or 'meridians' along which energy known as Qi (pronounced 'chee') flows.[5] Qi or energy underlies the balanced functioning in the body and when it becomes blocked or deficient we become unhealthy. The points are carefully chosen by the practitioner in order to disperse any blockages and to bring your Qi into a better balance (for more on Qi see Chapter 6). The more this balance is achieved and maintained, the healthier you become.

When I first saw acupuncture being practised I thought it looked very easy to do. I soon learned that this wasn't true.

Although it appears very simple from the outside, it takes years of in-depth study to learn where to place the needles in order to treat patients accurately and with care and sensitivity.

The study of acupuncture covers many components. These include how to correctly make a Chinese medicine diagnosis, how to recognise which points to use, how to locate the points, how to interact with people and how to insert the needles to the best effect. Although a Chinese medicine diagnosis uses a completely different paradigm from that of a Western diagnosis, practitioners also study Western medicine in order to understand when to refer and to understand the effects of medicinal drugs.

When choosing a practitioner it is important to ensure that you choose someone who is well qualified (see The British Acupuncture Council, Useful Addresses, p. 272). Professional acupuncturists who use the traditional style of treatment you will be reading about in this book have studied for at least three years in order to become competent practitioners. Some doctors and physiotherapists have taken longer courses in acupuncture, but most have taken short courses lasting only one or two weekends. Although they may be extremely competent physiotherapists or doctors this doesn't necessarily mean they have sufficient training in Chinese medicine. These practitioners will usually be trained to deal with a limited range of conditions and are unlikely to be treating the underlying cause of a condition, as would a professional practitioner.[6]

Diagnosing and treating with acupuncture

Acupuncture can treat a vast array of different illnesses. Sometimes when I am asked, 'What can it help?' I have to think hard before answering. This is not because I don't know what it *can* help but more because it is hard to say what it *can't* help. Its effects are wide-ranging and broad. Because acupuncture is holistic, it treats a patient's body, mind and emotions and deals with a whole range of acute and chronic problems.

Chinese medical treatment is different from that of Western medicine in many ways. When you are treated with Western medicine, your practitioner will usually concentrate on diagnosing and treating your outward signs and symptoms. In contrast, acupuncture recognises that all problems have an underlying cause. The practitioner aims to find and treat the root cause of your problem in order to alleviate your presenting condition. Dealing only with your signs and symptoms without dealing with the underlying cause tends to produce a temporary alleviation, but it won't last. Rather than considering whether acupuncture can help your signs and symptoms, your practitioner will probably ask, 'Can acupuncture help this person?'[7]

Your acupuncturist's diagnosis and treatment is different from that used by a practitioner of Western medicine, but this doesn't mean that acupuncture can't have a beneficial effect on many different 'named' illnesses. People come to treatment with a whole range of problems varying from headaches to gynaecological problems or from depression or anxiety to musculo-skeletal aches and pains.

Current research into acupuncture

Although practitioners know that acupuncture can treat a huge number of conditions, research is still 'proving' its effects. A report from the World Health Organization (WHO) in 2001 reviewed many clinical trials into the effects of acupuncture. Although it didn't cover every illness that acupuncture can treat, it did list 28 conditions that acupuncture has been proved to treat effectively and 63 where acupuncture has been shown to be effective but further proof is needed.

The 28 condition with the most compelling evidence in the WHO report were: adverse reactions to radiotherapy and/or chemotherapy, allergic rhinitis, bilary colic, depression, dysentery, dysmenorrhoea (period pains), acute epigastric pain, facial pain, headaches, hypertension, induction of labour, knee pain, low back pain, malposition of the foetus in pregnancy, morning sickness, nausea and vomiting, neck pain, pain in dentistry, post-operative pain, renal colic, rheumatoid arthritis, sciatica, arthritis of the shoulder, sprains, stroke and tennis elbow.

Some of the 63 conditions in the report where acupuncture has been shown to be effective but further proof is needed are: abdominal pain, acne vulgaris, alcohol dependence, bronchial asthma, cancer pain, cardiac neurosis, 'competition stress' syndrome, non-insulin-dependent diabetes, earache, eye pain, female infertility, facial spasm, fibro-myalgia, gallstones, gouty arthritis, herpes zoster (shingles), insomnia, labour pain, lactation deficiency, male sexual dysfunction, Menière's disease (severe attacks of dizziness and ringing in the ears), neurodermatitis, nosebleeds, obesity, opium, cocaine and heroin dependence, osteo-arthritis, polycystic ovary syndrome, post-operative convalescence, pre-menstrual syndrome, prostatitis, Raynaud's syndrome, recurrent lower urinary tract infection, retention of urine, schizophrenia, sore throat, spine pain, stiff neck, tobacco dependence, Tourette's syndrome, ulcerative colitis (inflammation and ulceration in the large intestine) and whooping cough.[8]

The WHO report relied heavily on Chinese studies but Western scientists prefer to use their own research. They start from the standpoint of having to prove an unknown therapy, whereas the Chinese, who have been using acupuncture for over 2,000 years, already believe that it works. Unfortunately the Western methods too have their drawbacks and have not always been the most appropriate for evaluating the benefits of acupuncture. Western scientists would recommend acupuncture for a much smaller list of conditions, mostly in the area of chronic pain, but additional research needs to be carried out as very few other illnesses have been thoroughly investigated so far.[9]

Why does acupuncture work?

Acupuncture first hit the headlines in the West when President Nixon visited China in 1972. A *New York Times* reporter, James Reston, had his appendix removed and wrote about the pain relief acupuncture had afforded him. Fully conscious Chinese patients undergoing major surgery with acupuncture anaesthesia were also seen on prime-time TV. Both the general public and the scientific community were fascinated. The race to find out how acupuncture worked was on. Because of this initial publicity, research was initially focused on the treatment of pain.

One discovery was that acupuncture stimulates the secretion of substances called endorphins. Endorphins are naturally occurring chemicals that are released in the brain. They have characteristics similar to pain-killing drugs such as morphine, and like morphine they kill pain. Various other neuro-chemicals (for example, serotonin and adenosine) are also now known to be involved in acupuncture's effects, particularly for pain, but also mood, immunity, hormones and other systems.[10]

Acupuncture works at both a local level, improving blood circulation and tissue repair, and throughout the body via nerve stimulation.[11] Studies have also found that acupuncture balances the autonomic nervous system. The autonomic nervous system regulates bodily functions that are not under our conscious control such as our heartbeat, intestinal movements and sweating. This in turn ensures that we can retain a healthy balance between relaxing and digesting our food or being prepared for action. Another study has shown that acupuncture affects the circulatory system and enables the blood vessels to constrict and dilate. This is thought to initiate healing by affecting the exchange of nutrients and the elimination of waste products within the small blood vessels or capillaries of the body. One exciting research development has been the use of powerful scanners to monitor brain activity before and after acupuncture. Needling appears to calm areas involved with pain and our response to pain, whilst activating those concerned with rest and relaxation.[12]

Although it is clear that acupuncture can have wide and varied physiological effects, these studies are still limited as they do not explain its many benefits. Perhaps we will never fully know why acupuncture works. This doesn't necessarily seem surprising when we consider that we still don't know why many other medicines (including a simple aspirin) affect our health! Some researchers have pointed out parallels between modern theories in physics and the important Chinese medicine notion of Qi or energy. Hopefully this will lead to acceptance of the fundamental concepts, medical and philosophical, underlying acupuncture.

I have seen so many patients benefit from acupuncture that I think one of the best ways of proving that it works is not to know why it works but rather to notice its effects. I would fully endorse the words of Bruce Pomeranz, who was one of the main researchers into endorphins and studies of how acupuncture works. He has noted, 'There is more to acupuncture than endorphins and the treatment of pain.'[13]

Acupuncture in practice

As a practitioner I see the powerful results of acupuncture every day in my own practice. I also see the effects of treatments carried out by students and colleagues. It is a common occurrence for patients to notice immediate changes after treatments and to comment on improvements such as their increased sense of well-being, greater energy, better balance in their temperature or a decrease in pain levels. Treatment also provides long-term improvements. It is these kinds of changes that make practising acupuncture so fascinating and rewarding for practitioners and so gratifying for patients.

In the next chapter you will meet some of these patients, who will tell their stories of how acupuncture has benefited them.

Summary

- Acupuncture is one of the fastest growing and most popular complementary therapies in the West.
- Because acupuncture is a holistic therapy it can treat a large range of different conditions that manifest in a patient's body, mind and spirit and may be acute or chronic.
- Much research has now been carried out into the effectiveness of acupuncture, but much remains to be done.
- Acupuncture is known to have many physiological effects particularly via neuro-chemicals such as secretions known as endorphins, which can kill pain. Subsequent studies have also shown many other beneficial effects of acupuncture.

2

Who Has Acupuncture?
What Does it Treat?

The benefits of acupuncture

In this chapter I will be introducing you to a range of people who've benefited from acupuncture and letting them tell you about their experiences of treatment. As the book progresses you will hear from these patients again, as well as hearing comments from other patients I've talked to while writing the book.

Who has acupuncture?

Young or old, male or female, anyone can benefit from acupuncture. Our college research mentioned in Chapter 1 defined a typical sample of patients. Approximately 67 per cent were women, their ages ranging from 10 to 88 years with an average age of 41 years. Most conditions treated were chronic and long term with over 80 per cent having had their complaint for at least a year and 50 per cent for over five years. Nearly three-quarters were affected at least once a day by their complaint.[1]

The research found that a majority (26.4 per cent) of patients had musculo-skeletal complaints (including arthritis and joint pain).[2] The next largest group (17 per cent) had general or unspecific symptoms such as general pain, weakness or tiredness, allergies, or viral or infectious diseases. The third most common group had psychological conditions (15.6 per cent). These included stress, depression, insomnia, poor memory or concentration, or substance abuse. Most patients had more than one complaint with the average number of complaints being two.[3]

Why do people embark on treatment?

Most people embark on treatment because others who have benefited from acupuncture have recommended it. There are also various other reasons. These include the recommendation of a general practitioner, an interest and fascination with acupuncture or Chinese philosophy or feeling ill enough to try anything!

Common conditions treated by acupuncture

The uniqueness of each patient

Although most patients come for treatment with a 'named' condition, an acupuncturist recognises that patients are individuals and that each has a unique experience of their problems. For example, there is a huge variation in the way patients experience headaches, digestive problems or feelings of depression or anxiety. On top of this there is an even greater number of physical, mental or emotional causes for these symptoms.

Categories of conditions

Acupuncture treats each person individually, but to ensure clarity I have divided the range of conditions it can treat into six broad categories, which are:

- Aches or pains
- Mental/emotional conditions
- Physical problems
- Acute infections and viral conditions
- Severe long-term chronic illnesses
- Preventative treatment

I will look at each of these in turn.

ACHES OR PAINS

This first category includes most musculo-skeletal conditions. This could be rheumatoid or osteo-arthritis or it could be pain affecting individual joints such as a backache, frozen shoulder, tennis or golfer's elbow, or wrist, hip, knee or ankle pain. These aches and pains may arise from a variety of causes including accidents or traumas and they may be long or short term, chronic or acute. This category also includes other pains such as headaches and migraines or fibro-myalgia.[4]

MENTAL/EMOTIONAL CONDITIONS

The second group is another, very different kind of pain – emotional pain. Patients might describe feeling depressed, having panic attacks or feeling anxious. They often find these internal states hard to describe. For example, patients have told me that they 'have lost confidence', 'feel despairing', 'feel jumpy and unable to settle inside', 'can't cope' or 'feel negative about everything'.

Acupuncture can help to stabilise people during a difficult but temporary or transitory phase in their lives such as bereavement, marriage break-up or when children leave home. Included in this section are people whose emotions are slightly unstable, causing symptoms such as moodiness or emotional swings, often with no obvious cause. In this case acupuncture can 'fine-tune' their energy so that they feel more stable.

This section also includes patients with more serious mental conditions such as schizophrenia or manic depression. Acupuncture can be very helpful for many of these conditions although its effectiveness varies according to how long the person has been ill, how severely she or he is ill and what medications are being taken.[5]

Finally, many patients have treatment for a physical condition and are then delighted to feel additional mental and/or emotional changes that affect their life in general.

PHYSICAL PROBLEMS

This group covers a broad range of conditions. They can be related to specific parts of the body and include digestive conditions, gynaecological problems, lung ailments, bowel disorders, urinary problems, circulatory disorders, ear, nose and throat conditions, eye problems, heart conditions and thyroid disorders. This is not an exhaustive list and many other complaints can be included. Many of these illnesses will be discussed in greater depth later in the book.

ACUTE INFECTIONS AND VIRAL CONDITIONS

Acute illnesses have a sudden onset and severe symptoms, but usually have a short duration. They include illnesses such as coughs and colds as well as other problems such as acute[6] bowel, stomach, ear or eye infections. Often these are not the patient's main complaint. More likely they have arisen and are treated during the period in which she or he is undergoing acupuncture treatment for other conditions. Also included in this group are acute viral conditions such as glandular fever, which can lead to a range of post-viral syndromes that are very common these days.

SEVERE LONG-TERM CHRONIC ILLNESSES

This category includes life-threatening illnesses suffered by those who are undergoing Western medical treatment at the same time as having acupuncture, for example patients with various forms of cancer or kidney disease. Also in this category are degenerative conditions such as multiple sclerosis, lupus, motor neurone disease and muscular dystrophy. Illnesses requiring replacement drugs such as diabetes (insulin), pernicious anaemia (vitamin B12) or Addison's disease (cortico-steroid drugs) also come into this category.

Some of the conditions in this group may overlap with those in other categories, especially those in the 'physical conditions' section. I have put them in their own separate section, however, as this group includes more severe conditions.

PREVENTATIVE TREATMENT

Many patients have acupuncture in order to remain healthy. Some of my patients come to treatment because they are merely curious about it, others because, although they have no 'named' condition, they have heard that acupuncture can positively enhance their health. Many other patients begin acupuncture treatment with a 'named' condition. Once this has been cured they continue to be treated every one to three months in order to stay well. This can be compared to giving a car a regular service in order to keep it in good condition. Consequently it has fewer breakdowns and does more miles to the gallon than a car that has been 'run into the ground' by its owner.

The different types of patients of helped by acupuncture

As well as choosing a selection of patients receiving treatment for each of the above groups of conditions, I have included summaries of research into these conditions.

The patients below all volunteered to speak to me about their treatment. I have changed their names to maintain confidentiality. Each patient has been helped by treatment in different ways and for different conditions. One patient, Craig, has had treatment for his rheumatoid arthritis while another, Jenny, became very anxious around the time of her exams at university. Yet another patient, Sarah, came because of her asthma, Samantha had a post-viral condition and Francesca had the support of acupuncture while she recovered from a mastectomy. Finally, Josie came with a fertility problem but has continued to have treatment in order to keep well – her daughter is now seven.

Most of these patients were treated by third-year acupuncture students at the College of Integrated Chinese Medicine UK under my supervision, or were my own patients. One patient, Samantha, was treated by a close colleague.

We'll now meet some of these patients.

Craig

Craig is 50 and married, with two grown-up children. He runs his own successful business. He came for treatment for rheumatoid arthritis four years ago and I supervised his treatment in the student clinic. This is what he told me about his treatment.

THE PROGRESS OF ARTHRITIS

'The arthritis was painful and scary. It started when I was about 31 or 32, very suddenly, over the period of a week. It started with a little ache in the heel of one hand and within the week I couldn't do up my shirt buttons. I could only release my finger joints by forcibly straightening them. Within a short time my knees, elbows and wrists were all hurting. It was agony to walk. In spite of hospital treatment nothing changed for 15 years. I took many medications and also had massive doses of aspirin at first. All I was offered besides these drugs was a neck brace or things to support the joints. I was in limbo. I had exceptional pain, limited movement and was waking up most nights unable to get up and walk to the loo. I can remember feeling as if I had huge stones stuck in my shoes when I walked. I was pretty depressed about it.'

GOING FOR TREATMENT

'I went for treatment because I knew someone who was an acupuncture student and I knew she needed a patient. I thought acupuncture should be interesting and I wasn't doing anything so I thought I'd give it a whirl. I had needles in various parts of my body, especially my arms. There was no sensation of the needles entering the body but I could feel the sensation of the needles once they were in. This could be strong but was not painful. It was surprising, as these were sensations I'd never had before.'

THE RESULTS OF TREATMENT

'The result of treatment is that I've now literally "thrown down my crutches and can walk"! It's astonishing. I get regular sleep and if I wake up a bit stiff in the morning, within minutes it's gone. I'm not on drugs now as I don't feel I need to take any. I get some pain occasionally but very little. There were big changes at first, then smaller ones as I progressed and I now have treatment every six weeks to two months to keep well. It took four or five months for my hands to get completely better.

'I feel happier in myself having had acupuncture and I have faith in acupuncture as a general means of treatment. I'd probably turn to it as a method of treatment if I had any illness. If I'd stuck with Western medicine I think I'd still be as bad as I was before. It's changed my life and for me it's absolutely amazing.'

Recent research into the effects of acupuncture in the treatment of pain

Craig is just one of many people with musculo-skeletal problems who have been helped by acupuncture. In a review of acupuncture trials the World Health Organization found that acupuncture can help many different musculo-skeletal problems. They found that it not only alleviates pain but also increases mobility and may bring about a permanent cure where muscular problems have increased joint pain. Research has been carried out into the effect of acupuncture on neck pain, peri-arthritis of the shoulder, fibro-myalgia, tennis elbow, low back pain, sciatica and osteo-arthritis with knee pain. It consistently has favourable results. It has also been found to help in the treatment of rheumatoid arthritis and to relieve pain, decrease inflammation and benefit the immune system.[7] Western medical researchers also endorse acupuncture for treating chronic pain.[8]

Jenny

Jenny was 22 when she came to the student clinic for treatment. Below she describes what she experienced.

BECOMING UNWELL

'I had been anxious since I was a child and was always aware of what people thought of me and tried to be good at school. I didn't slip out of line much. I then got stressed in my final year at university. I wasn't eating well and I got panicky and didn't cope with the stress very well. The weather has a huge effect on me too and cold and damp made me worse. A friend's mum had already gone to the clinic and told me I should go. I'd tried everything else really so I thought I'd try it.'

THE REASONS FOR TREATMENT

'I went for treatment for two reasons, because of the anxiety and because I had a skin condition. I often had a vague feeling of unease and could get really quite anxious in certain situations. For instance, if I made a mistake at work I'd feel everyone was watching me. I'd then feel my heart beating fast and I'd become short of breath and find it difficult to concentrate. Sometimes I'd feel a low-grade anxiety for no reason. The anxiety made it hard for me to get off to sleep – I never slept deeply and small noises would easily wake me. The more stressed I felt the more difficult it was to sleep and it could take up to three hours for me to get off to sleep. I also had eczema resulting from this. I went to the doctor and he gave me steroid creams for the eczema but it didn't make it go away. It got to a point where it was all over my body. Herbs didn't help either. The doctor just gave me a stronger cream. None of it worked. If something rubbed against my skin it would get worse and it would flare up after a shower.'

HAVING A TREATMENT

'Sometimes the needles were left in and at other times they were removed almost immediately. I feel completely fine about the needles. There are sometimes quite nice feelings like a muscle tugging then relaxing. There's nothing unpleasant or that really hurts. After treatments I really felt different. I often felt relaxed, sleepy and floating.'

THE RESULTS OF TREATMENT

'I've now had about eight treatments. I feel a lot calmer and can cope much better. I've also been much brighter in myself and have more strength and energy, which means I can do more. My sleeping is now completely fine – in fact I'm sleeping like a baby! Before I couldn't handle it if I didn't have enough sleep, now I can cope a lot better. The eczema cleared up almost immediately from my arms and legs. I'd expected acupuncture to be all about my physical problem rather than the emotional issues although I can see now that it's where it all started.'

Research into acupuncture for mental–emotional problems

Acupuncture was very helpful to Jenny's underlying anxiety and consequently helped her skin condition. As well as treating anxiety and panic attacks it can also been shown to be effective in the treatment of other mental–emotional disorders such as depression. In research into its effect on depression, the World Health Organization has found that acupuncture compares favourably with medicinal drugs, with the added benefit that it has no side effects. Research has also shown that acupuncture can be more effective in the treatment of schizophrenia than chlorpromazine, one of the main drugs used in its treatment.[9]

Western researchers acknowledge that acupuncture compares favourably with medication for depression[10] and schizophrenia[11] but as yet have held back from endorsing it because of the paradoxical results from trials investigating the strength of the placebo effect[12].

Sarah

Sarah is 56 and a retired nurse. I find it impossible not to love her bright and cheerful disposition. In fact she was so good-natured that she was nicknamed 'Sunny Sarah' by her boss.

THE REASON FOR TREATMENT

'I went for treatment with asthma but I also had loads of other things wrong with me – arthritis in the knees and hands, psoriasis, and emotional problems.

'The asthma came on when I gave up smoking. I was really ill with a bad chest and it turned to bronchial asthma. I think it was the shock to my system of giving everything up. I came from a family of smokers and was naughty. I'd smoked since I was a little girl of 11 – I wouldn't go to school unless my mum gave me a cigarette!

'I decided to have treatment because I didn't think conventional medicine was doing me any good. I had a friend who had had good results from acupuncture – she'd had a bad back that had improved and she said she thought it could help me too. At the time of starting treatment I was on four inhalers, taking four puffs a day. In between I regularly took steroids when I was really bad.'

THE EXPERIENCE OF TREATMENT

'When I first went for treatment it was like a weight had been lifted from me. Although the asthma came on after I gave up smoking I think emotional problems played a big part too. I appreciated the fact that my acupuncturist spent time with me and it was important that she listened to me.

'The needles don't bother me at all. I've had them in my feet, legs, arms and wrists, only a few at a time. They don't hurt but there is a sensation. I'm not scared of them and I don't find them uncomfortable at all.

'I often go to sleep during the treatment as it's very relaxing and very calming. It makes me feel very good. I often feel as if I'm floating on air afterwards. I could run a marathon – after I've had a sleep first though!'

THE RESULTS OF TREATMENT

'My chest isn't perfect yet but I haven't had steroids since I've been coming for treatment. I still use some inhalers but have cut right down. The pains in my knees and hands have also completely gone and I feel much happier too. I love having treatment and can't wait for the next one.'

Current research into acupuncture in the treatment of asthma

Many practitioners find that acupuncture can be very helpful in the treatment of asthma. According to the World Health Organization, there are conflicting results from trials in treating bronchial asthma with acupuncture; however, it does say that the majority of reports suggest such treatment is very effective.[13]

Samantha

Samantha is 30 years old and is chatty and full of life. Having spoken to her recently, it is hard to imagine how ill she was before she had treatment from one of my colleagues.

BECOMING ILL

'I had what was called ME, a post-viral syndrome.[14] Before getting ill I'd always exercised and been healthy. I didn't smoke or drink excessively and I was quite fit. Then I had glandular fever at 18. I also had a stressful job and was studying law, which wasn't right for me. At that time I bottled things up and didn't talk about it. With all the stress I think my immune system was affected. The ME came and went a number of times but I always went back to a stressful job, which I wasn't finding fulfilling. Finally it struck again at 26 and it didn't get better.'

THE MAIN SYMPTOMS

'There was no tiredness like it. It was like my blood had been replaced with lead and like I had a big fat suit on all the time with heavy weights hanging from it. I used to like to go swimming but even picking up my swimming bag was a strain. By the time I got to the pool I could hardly swim a length.

'My digestion was dreadful too. Whenever I ate I came out in a sweat. I would be dripping with sweat. It was like a hot flush. I had no interest in anything. There was a lack of understanding about it. Instead of being sympathetic, people would keep asking "Are you better?" It was frustrating because I wasn't.'

THE DECISION TO HAVE TREATMENT

'I'd been open-minded about any complementary therapy but wasn't too sure about going to acupuncture. I'd tried homeopathy for a year and had seen a nutritionist but still wasn't better. My morale was low as nothing had worked. I'd been recommended to go to my practitioner by my GP so I thought I'd try it, but I didn't have much hope.'

TREATMENT AND ITS EFFECTS

'At first I felt very tired afterwards but it was different – a nice tiredness. I had weekly treatments at that time. Now I don't feel tired after treatment and it gives me extra fuel and a lift. It now lasts me for a whole month and it's been constant. Some of the first signs that I was improving were that I could go out shopping and not be knocked out or could go out and be OK the next day.

'I think it really helped my mind too. My interest came back. For example, I could cook a meal and wanted to pick up a newspaper or watch TV. Acupuncture changed the impact things had on me. I felt more positive and I stopped stressing about whether I could cope with things. Before I would be wiped out the rest of the week. I had to stop comparing myself to my old self though.

'I started college this week. For me who lay on the settee for five years it was a real achievement. I still can't drink alcohol and if I have busy day I have to be careful about how much I do the next day, but I'm so much better and I now go for treatment every month.'

Research into strengthening the immune system

Samantha responded very well to acupuncture treatment. Although it doesn't help in every case I have seen many others with post-viral syndrome also have successful results. A report from the World Health Organization stated that research has found that acupuncture can stimulate the immune system, especially when it is used with other medical therapies for treating infections, but more research clearly needs to be carried out in this area.[15]

A recent Chinese analysis found acupuncture to be effective for chronic fatigue syndrome.[16] As yet there have not been any substantial studies in the West on chronic fatigue syndrome but there is evidence that acupuncture can benefit the immune system across a variety of different conditions.[17]

Francesca

At the age of 52 Francesca is now embarking on training to become an acupuncturist herself. This follows the support she had from treatment in the student clinic while she was undergoing chemotherapy.

THE REASON FOR TREATMENT

'When I came for treatment I was having chemotherapy. I'd been diagnosed with breast cancer and had had a mastectomy.

When I was first diagnosed I really thought I'd die, but once I'd had the mastectomy I was told the results were good. The chemotherapy was hell. I felt sick and ill. I couldn't walk. I lost my hair. It was hell on earth. If it came back there's no way I'd go through that again. It was awful.'

BECOMING ILL

'I think the breast cancer was waiting to happen although I didn't see it at the time. I had a marriage break-up at 37, was on a terrible diet and I was taking HRT. Also people in my family had had it.

'I didn't go to acupuncture saying, "Oh, it's what I want." I said, "I'll try anything," and the opportunity was there. I had no preconceptions. I was in the middle of chemotherapy so I wasn't thinking straight and I had no confidence it would help me.'

THE EFFECTS OF TREATMENT

'Acupuncture definitely helped me cope with chemotherapy much better. I had acupuncture after the fourth chemotherapy session. From then onwards I was able to cope with it. I was flat on my back for the first three sessions. I think the effect of the chemotherapy could have been even worse for sessions four, five and six but instead it was a lot more bearable. Life in general was a lot more bearable. I didn't sleep as much and there was not such a battle going on in my stomach, so I was less nauseous.

'I now think that if I'd had treatment before I wouldn't have fallen ill and I'd have been more robust. I had the extra energy to cope with what was going on. I also wish I'd had it during my marriage break-up, as I know it would have helped. I felt different from treatment and there was nothing else going on that could have done it.'

Research into the treatment of cancer patients with acupuncture

Acupuncture is quite widely used by cancer sufferers, particularly for helping to moderate the side effects of chemo- and radiotherapy, such as nausea and vomiting, hot flushes, dry mouth and lowered immunity.[18] Stimulation of acupuncture points has also been shown to be effective for the management of therapy-related adverse events in patients with breast cancer.[19] In pain arising from cancer it has been shown to provide immediate relief similar to codeine and pethidine, with a more marked effect after use for two months.

Josie

Josie is a teacher who initially came for treatment for infertility. When she started having treatment she had two children but couldn't conceive a third. She now has three. She continues to come for treatment to ensure she stays well and has been having treatment for about nine years. This is what she says about her experience of treatment.

WHY ACUPUNCTURE?

'A friend had benefited from treatment and said the practitioner was a caring and sensitive person. I wanted to get pregnant and I thought, "I want to try it." Before treatment I didn't think too much about it. I might have had a little apprehension but someone explained what to expect and I thought I fancied it. It was a gut instinct that it was right for me.'

GOING TO TREATMENT

'I didn't really have a complaint but I did have trouble getting pregnant and didn't want to take drugs. I wanted to get pregnant and be healthy. I'd had two miscarriages and since then had been trying to conceive for two years. I started acupuncture in

September, then my mum died in December so treatment took a different turn and helped me through that difficult time. I would never have come for that reason, but it really helped to support me.'

THE EFFECTS OF TREATMENT

'I look forward to the treatment and I even love watching the needles go in! I take an interest in what's going on. The needle sensation is like a dull ache and sometimes there's a pleasant feeling of release.

'When I have treatment it's like an instant tranquilliser. Sometimes I have to shut my eyes – everything is more relaxed. It's like feeling drugged without being woozy. There have been times when I've been walking home on a cloud.

'During my pregnancy the treatment kept my blood pressure down. I was 11 years older than when I'd had my first and second children but my blood pressure was lower. I called her my alternative baby! It was really important for me to know that my practitioner was at hand to give treatment if the baby hadn't engaged. I was a prime candidate for intervention and I was so relaxed during the pregnancy and labour. My daughter is now seven!

'Long-term treatment has affected me in loads of ways. I generally feel healthier by a long chalk. I never get colds any more and it has helped me to relax and take things more in my stride. I have acupuncture regularly – about every six weeks – as it keeps me on top of things both mentally and physically. I recommend it all the time and my husband, who now also has it, calls it "magic". When you desperately need it, it's potent stuff. If I didn't have it I know I wouldn't be as well as I am today.'

Research into the effect of acupuncture during pregnancy and labour

Josie now uses acupuncture in order to stay healthy but she originally came to treatment because she wanted to become pregnant. Like Josie, many people with fertility problems gain benefit from acupuncture.

Reviews of the literature on acupuncture for fertility suggest that it may act by reducing stress, increasing blood flow to the reproductive organs and improving neurological and hormonal control of reproductive processes.[20] Thus acupuncture can normalise ovulation and the menstrual cycle and benefit fertility. Women who incorporate acupuncture into their in-vitro fertilisation IVF treatment may be more likely to become pregnant than those who use IVF alone.[21]

The World Health Organization has also found acupuncture to be helpful in other areas of pregnancy and labour such as morning sickness, prevention of miscarriage and to correct an abnormal foetal position.[22]

Summary

- A vast spectrum of patients from all walks of life and with many different conditions are successfully treated with acupuncture.
- Although most patients come for treatment with a 'named' condition, an acupuncturist recognises that patients are individuals and that each experiences their problems in their own unique way.
- Acupuncture treats each person individually, but the range of conditions it can treat falls into six broad categories:
  - Aches or pains
  - Mental/emotional conditions
  - Physical problems
  - Acute infections and viral conditions

- Severe long-term chronic illnesses
- Preventative treatment
- Research into the effect of treatment is beginning to prove that acupuncture works. Acupuncturists have known of its benefits for thousands of years of course!

3

What Is it Like to Have Treatment? Needles and Moxibustion

Finding out about you and your health

New patients usually have a number of questions and many of these are centred on the needles, for example: 'Do the needles hurt?' 'How are they sterilised?' 'How many needles will you use?' and 'How long will the needles be left in?' I'll answer all of these important questions and many others in this chapter.

Before going any further, however, let me assure you that acupuncture is not about needles alone. After you've started having acupuncture any worries about needles are likely to fade as you relax and enjoy the experience of the treatment and the resulting health benefits.

The importance of rapport

Acupuncturists come in all shapes and sizes, so there will be some variation in how each one relates to you. What they all have in common, however, is that they value the therapeutic relationship and want to have a good rapport with you. They know that the connection between you is a vital key that enables you to open up and talk. If you like and trust your practitioner, you can relax. If you don't feel at ease, the treatment is less likely to go well. Although treatment is not dependent on how well you communicate (it works on children and animals, as you'll see later), good rapport can accelerate its progress.

The first consultation and subsequent treatment

The diagnosis is carried out at the first visit so this session takes longer than the subsequent treatments. During this first consultation, your acupuncturist will ask you lots of questions about yourself. A diagnosis is literally the foundation of treatment. By finding out about you and your health, your practitioner can decide on how best to treat you. The resulting treatment plan forms the basis from which your acupuncturist carries out the subsequent treatments.

I describe the process of diagnosis in greater depth in Chapter 8. For now I'll give you a brief summary of what's involved and then tell you more about how you'll be likely to experience each treatment.

The diagnosis

Although your acupuncturist will ask you quite a few questions during your diagnosis, her or his main intention is to listen to what you have to say. What she or he asks, however, won't require huge feats of memory from you. As well as asking you about your signs and symptoms, your acupuncturist will be diagnosing the underlying cause of your problem. Everyone's diagnosis is different and your treatments are made to measure especially for you.

You'll be asked questions about your main complaint and your general health. General health involves such things as your sleep, your appetite and your perspiration. Other questions may seem to have less relevance to your health but are no less important. For example, your acupuncturist may ask you about the tastes you prefer, when your energy is better or worse or whether you prefer hot or cold weather. Although these may seem irrelevant, they enable your practitioner to make a holistic and individual diagnosis of you.

As well as asking you these questions, your practitioner will also carry out a physical examination. During this, she or he will feel your pulses and look at your tongue.

The sequence of the first consultation

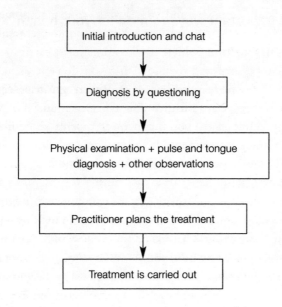

Initial introduction and chat

Diagnosis by questioning

Physical examination + pulse and tongue diagnosis + other observations

Practitioner plans the treatment

Treatment is carried out

Sometimes the first treatment doesn't take place until the second visit.

In the treatment room

Once you've had a diagnosis you will be ready for a treatment. At the start of each treatment your acupuncturist will find out how you are progressing. She or he will then gather more information by feeling pulses on your wrist and looking at your tongue. Pulse and tongue diagnosis are used to assess your overall health. Your practitioner will also observe your facial colour and other signs and will then decide on treatment principles. The treatment principles are the guidelines for treatment and they will enable your acupuncturist to choose the best points to achieve a better balance in your health. Treatment is then carried out using needles and/or moxibustion.

Some important ways to monitor your health

PULSE DIAGNOSIS

You may be surprised to know that you don't have just one pulse that can be felt on your wrist. Rather you have 12, each of which is associated with a different Organ and has distinct qualities. While studying acupuncture, students practise taking and recording pulses in order to become sensitive to them. Pulse diagnosis forms an important part of both diagnosis and treatment. Having felt your pulses during the diagnosis and at the beginning of treatment, your acupuncturist might feel them again a number of times as treatment progresses. This is because the pulses alter during the course of treatment and enable your acupuncturist to monitor how well your treatment is progressing. I will discuss this further in Chapter 9.

TONGUE DIAGNOSIS

Observing the tongue is a very sophisticated method of diagnosis. It works because the tongue is one of the few places where the inside of the body can be seen on the outside. Your acupuncturist will look at your tongue during your initial visit and at each subsequent treatment. As treatment progresses your tongue body and coating will gradually change, indicating that you are becoming healthier. Different areas of the tongue are associated with the different Organs (see diagram below) and your practitioner will be looking for any cracks, spots, or different colours in these areas.

Like pulse diagnosis, I will be discussing the tongue in greater depth in Chapter 8.

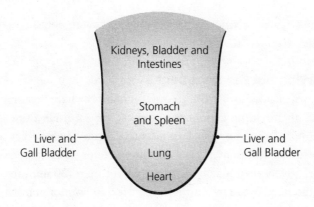

Kidneys, Bladder and
Intestines

Stomach
and Spleen

Liver and
Gall Bladder

Liver and
Gall Bladder

Lung

Heart

OBSERVING FACIAL COLOUR AND OTHER SIGNS

As well as assessing your pulse and tongue your acupuncturist will also make other observations. These include looking at your facial colour, listening to your voice tone and assessing your general emotional balance.

Planning the treatment

The slant of treatment varies according to your changing needs. Your feedback and your practitioner's observations are crucial when establishing the direction of treatment. This is especially true in the early stages – it's important that the patient and practitioner work as a team.

To clarify how treatment needs to progress, acupuncturists might ask themselves questions, such as: 'How well is this patient improving?' 'Which part of my treatment plan should now take precedence?' 'Is the treatment reaching every level of the patient?'

Later, as the diagnosis becomes established, your acupuncturist will still need to gather accurate information about you. Your relationship with your acupuncturist is vital in order to do this. The direction of the treatment can then be changed according to your needs.

Once your practitioner has planned the treatment, she or he is ready to insert the needles.

Carrying out the treatment

You will normally lie on a couch when you have treatment, although for some acupuncture points, for example those on your back, you may need to sit on a chair. The needles are sometimes withdrawn only a few seconds after insertion. Alternatively they may be left in place for up to 20 minutes.

If the needles are left in they won't feel uncomfortable. Most people feel happy to relax once they are inserted and sometimes even go to sleep. As Sarah said when her needles were left in, 'I often go to sleep during the treatment as it's very relaxing and very calming. It makes me feel very good. I often feel as if I'm floating on air afterwards.'

After removing the needles at the end of treatment your practitioner will usually feel your pulses to check that treatment has created greater harmony and balance in your Qi. How you feel after treatment varies. Some people feel no immediate change, others a sense of well-being and vitality. I will talk more about that later in this chapter.

The sequence of the treatment sessions

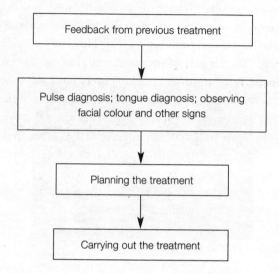

Feedback from previous treatment

Pulse diagnosis; tongue diagnosis; observing facial colour and other signs

Planning the treatment

Carrying out the treatment

Your questions about needles

What are the needles like?

Patients are often reassured to discover that acupuncture needles are very fine. They are different from the first needles that were used over 2,000 years ago. These were made from bamboo or stone. Later on iron needles were used. Gold and silver needles have been used too. Nowadays needles are most commonly made from stainless steel. This gives them certain important qualities. They are impossible to break, very flexible, and will not rust.

Acupuncture needles are very different from hypodermic needles. Hypodermics are used to inject substances into the body, so they have a hollow centre and are relatively thick. It is important to note that no substances are ever injected through an acupuncture needle and therefore the needle is solid. Acupuncture needles also look very different from hypodermic needles. They have a coiled handle, a thin gauge and a very sharp point – so that they can be inserted painlessly.

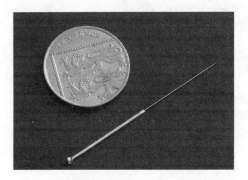

The length of the needles vary according to which area of the body needs to be treated. Some needles are half an inch long (approximately 13mm), some an inch (25.5mm), while others are longer.

Ancient Chinese doctors – *Huang Fu Mi* and his medical texts

Huang Fu Mi (pronounced 'Hwang Foo Mee') was born in the year AD 215. He became a doctor partly because of his desire to help his mother who was paralysed. Later on in his life he became ill himself and suffered from a form of rheumatism that severely disabled him.

He wrote an important medical text called the *Zhen Jiu Jia Yi Jing* (pronounced 'Jen Jee-ewe Je-ar Ye Jing'), which means the Compendium of Acupuncture and Moxibustion. In this book he describes many aspects of acupuncture treatment, explaining where the acupuncture points are located and what patterns of illness they can treat. He also wrote clearly about the theory of Chinese medicine and described various treatment methods. His book forms the basis for many modern Chinese medical textbooks.

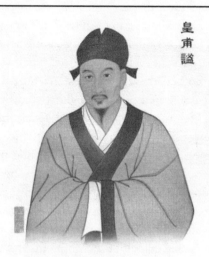

How are needles sterilised?

Acupuncturists always employ single use pre-sterilised disposable needles when treating patients. Each needle is disposed of in a sharps box after use. This ensures that no infection can be transmitted between patients, and that each patient is treated with the highest standard of care and cleanliness.

All qualified acupuncturists have been trained to use impeccable standards of hygiene when carrying out needle technique and they abide by a stringent code of safe practice, which has been laid down and is policed by their professional body.[1] Health and safety checks are also made by the local authority.

To date there have been no known incidents of infections being transmitted by members of the British Acupuncture Council, the largest professional acupuncture body in the UK.

Do the needles hurt?

This is the most common question that I am asked by new patients. Everyone is understandably anxious about pain. It is such an important question that it's probably best to recap on what some of the patients you met in Chapter 2 had to say about it.

Josie said, 'The needle sensation is like a dull ache and sometimes there's a pleasant feeling of release.' Sarah told me, 'The needles don't bother me at all. They don't hurt but there is a sensation. I'm not scared of them; I don't find them uncomfortable at all.' Jenny's comment was, 'I feel completely fine about the needles. There are sometimes quite nice feelings like a muscle tugging then relaxing. There's nothing unpleasant or that really hurts.' Finally Craig said, 'There was no sensation of the needles entering the body but I could feel the sensation of the needles once they were in. This could be strong but was not painful. It was surprising, as these were sensations I'd never had before.' You'll notice that all of these patients talk about a sensation arising from a needle but not pain.[2]

The acupuncturist first inserts the needle to penetrate the skin using a 'guide tube'. This is a sterilised tube which keeps the needle clean as well as ensuring a smooth and painless insertion. The needle is then guided to the correct point depth.

Once the needle has reached the correct depth the patient should feel a slight sensation as the needle contacts the Qi. This feeling is known as 'deqi'. Deqi is not unpleasant and is sometimes felt as a drawing sensation which the practitioner experiences as the needle being pulled, 'like catching a fish'. Its sensation can either be an ache, numbness, a tingling or a sensation of heat. This feeling only lasts for a couple of seconds. Very occasionally you may feel slightly more sensation from the needles. If this happens it is often a sign that there is more blockage of the Qi and a stronger needle manipulation has been required.

How many needles are used at each treatment?

In general, four to ten needles are used per treatment, but the number varies according to your condition and the strength of your Qi. For example, your acupuncturist will use more needles if you have an acute condition involving a block rather than a chronic one. Your practitioner will also vary the number of needles according to the strength of your constitution – if you have a more fragile constitution you may require fewer needles than if you have a stronger one.

If you have a musculo-skeletal problem, a larger number of needles may sometimes be used in a localised area to move any obstruction in order to free the joint. Craig, who had rheumatoid arthritis, for example, needed more needles than Samantha, who had a post-viral syndrome, or Josie, who now has preventative constitutional treatment.

How deep do the needles go?

The depth to which your acupuncturist inserts a needle will vary according to your size and the area being treated. The most common depths vary from a quarter to half an inch (approximately 6–13mm). A point that is on a non-fleshy area of the body, such as a toe, will penetrate to only about one-tenth of an inch (approximately 2mm). On fleshy areas such as the buttocks, where points are commonly used for hip pain, the needles will go in deeper and can be inserted to at least one and a half inches (approximately 38mm). The amount of sensation felt from the needle is not linked to the depth of the points. Some points that are nearer the surface can create more sensation than ones deeper inside the body.

Will the needles make me bleed?

You may be surprised to find that it is extremely unusual for acupuncture needles to draw blood during a treatment. People often expect that any penetration of the skin will result in bleeding, but acupuncture needles are so fine that they won't normally pierce blood vessels. On some rare occasions a small drop of blood is drawn and a tiny bruise can appear. This will have no detrimental effect on the treatment and is nothing to worry about.

Moxibustion

Needles are not the only form of treatment acupuncturists use. Another form of treatment is called moxibustion (also known as 'moxa'). Moxa has been used alongside acupuncture throughout Chinese history; in fact, the two words that the Chinese use for this therapy are *zhen* and *jiu* (pronounced 'jen' and 'jee-uw'). *Zhen* means 'needles' and *jiu* means 'moxa'. Because needles are so intriguing they often receive more publicity than moxa. Moxa, however, is also a very interesting and effective treatment, as you will now see.

Moxibustion is carried out by burning a herb close to or on your body in order to warm and nourish your Qi. The herb used is *Artemisia vulgaris latiflora*, which is similar to our native mugwort, a weed that grows by the roadside.

The leaves of *Artemisia vulgaris latiflora* are dried and pulverised, to be turned into what is called moxa 'wool' or moxa 'punk'. Its light brown colour and softness resembles a mixture between wool and cardboard. Its unimpressive appearance is deceptive, however. When it is lit, it has an unmistakable aroma that fills the treatment room. It is this pungent odour, as well as the warmth given off by the burning of the herb, that provides its healing effect. Traditionally moxa was first used in northern parts of China, where the climate is colder.

Why moxa is used in treatment

Moxa is used for two main reasons. First, it warms you up when you have a condition that is particularly 'cold' in its nature. Such conditions might vary from a painful joint to a cold lower abdomen or an aching, cold lower back. In these cases the moxa produces a strong heat with a penetrating effect. This can 'drive' the cold from the body and, over time, ease the condition completely. Josie, for example, was treated with moxa on her lower abdomen in order to warm the area and help her fertility. Craig was treated with moxa on his joints.

Second, moxa can be used to nourish your Qi and Blood. If you feel generally depleted in energy, have a weakness in one or more Organs or feel susceptible to cold weather then moxa can often add to the beneficial effects of the needles. In this case it will warm and strengthen your energy.

Methods of using moxa

Moxa can be used as a stick or as small cones, heated on the end of a needle or burnt in a special 'moxa box'.

A moxa stick looks similar to a cigar. After the stick is lit it is held over a point or moved over an area of your body to nourish and warm it. It is often used on large areas that need to be warmed. Common areas are the lower back, lower abdomen or stomach, although it can also warm a joint or a channel.

Moxa cones are placed on specific acupuncture points. A cone is individually lit and allowed to smoulder. It is then removed as soon as it becomes warm. Three to seven moxa cones are usually used on one point although sometimes more are required. This method of treatment is most often used if your energy generally needs to be nourished.

Moxa on a needle is beneficial when you require deep heat at a special point, for instance if you have a painful and cold joint such as a shoulder or hip. The moxa is attached to the handle of the needle and is lit. The sensation of warmth travels down the needle and penetrates deep inside the body. This can be very comforting and healing and clear the cold from the area.

Finally, the moxa box, like the moxa stick, can be used to heat up a large area of the body. This may be the lower back, abdomen or stomach. The moxa wool is placed in the special box and left to smoulder, creating a large area of heat. For example, a moxa box can be extremely comforting for patients with period pains due to a 'cold lower abdomen'. One patient told me, 'I once had period pains which were really severe and cramping. When my acupuncturist used a moxa box on the area, it cleared the pain miraculously. She then gave me a moxa stick to use at home. It felt very comforting to know I had something to control the pain.'

When moxa is not used

Although moxibustion can benefit a large number of patients it is sometimes contra-indicated. For instance, it is not usually used if you are already very hot or have a 'hot condition'. A hot condition can be indicated by symptoms such as profuse bleeding, like nosebleeds or heavy periods, or by inflammations or infections.

More about treatment

How does the practitioner know a treatment has worked?

There are a number of signs that let your practitioner know the treatment has been effective. I mentioned earlier in the chapter that your acupuncturist feels 12 pulses on the your wrist to diagnose the strength and quality of your Qi. During the course of a treatment your pulses change and your practitioner will expect to feel a general improvement in the pulse qualities by the end of treatment. This indicates that your treatment is progressing in a positive way. For more on this see Chapter 8.

Your acupuncturist may also observe small changes in your facial colour or voice tone, a change in your posture or even a renewed sparkle in your eyes. A shine in the eyes is always a good sign. It indicates that your spirit is strong and settled. If your eyes look clearer after a treatment this shows that a positive change is occurring in your spirit. Along with this, your acupuncturist may also notice if there is an improvement in your overall mood and well-being, showing that a change is occurring from deep inside.

How will I feel after treatment?

Some patients, like Craig who had rheumatoid arthritis, experience immediate improvement after treatment. He told me: 'I was euphoric after my first treatment, it was so nice I bought a new fishing rod! I went out saying "That was good. I think I'll buy something." I felt like I was enriched – it was a huge switch from being negative to positive.'

Other patients can take longer to notice changes and a number of treatments are required to create an effect which eventually becomes noticeable. Francesca, who was having chemotherapy, said, 'Not much happened at first, then later I felt better after a few days. I felt better but it was more the build-up over time and I definitely felt more able to cope with the chemotherapy.'

By about the fourth to the sixth treatment you will normally have felt some improvement and know that treatment is working. It is important that you and your practitioner continually monitor how treatment is progressing. Each patient's health improves in a different way (remember what I said earlier – we are all unique!).

Frequency of treatment

How often you come for treatment depends on your condition. You may start off having weekly treatments. As your condition improves, the treatment will then take place less often. You may then come for treatment every two weeks, and subsequently every three or four weeks. Once you are better, you can be checked at regular intervals to keep yourself well and you may even gain further improvement. For example, Josie and Craig still have treatment on a regular basis. Jenny, on the other hand, stopped treatment after her symptoms got better.

If you start with an extremely acute condition, such as an acute pain, infection or other injury, you might initially have sessions every day or every other day.

How long will it take?

The first consultation will usually last up to one and a half hours and the subsequent treatments anything from half an hour to one hour. Some practitioners take longer, others take less time. You can ask your practitioner how long the consultation and treatments are likely to take when you phone to arrange an appointment.

Do I have to believe in it for it to work?

People can benefit from acupuncture whether they believe in it or not. Although it is always helpful to come to treatment with a certain amount of confidence in it, many people who are initially sceptical are delighted by its positive results. I'm continually surprised that it is often the doubters who end up becoming acupuncture's most enthusiastic proponents.

How long will a course of treatment take?

Each patient takes a different length of time to get better. An acute symptom can often be cleared in one to four treatments in quick succession, but chronic problems usually take longer.

An illness that began in early childhood is bound to take longer to heal than one that started only recently. For some people who have been ill since childhood it may be months or even years before treatment is fully completed. For others only a few sessions are needed. As a rule of thumb practitioners often say it takes a month of treatment for every year you have been ill.

Can I still have preventative treatment if I don't have a complaint?

If you have no symptoms this doesn't matter. Your acupuncturist can still observe your pulses, tongue, facial colour and emotional balance to assess your Qi. Treatment can then harmonise any imbalances that have started to occur. I've known some people come to their first treatment with no main complaint, but this is rare. Preventative treatments are usually given when patients have recovered from their illness and wish to continue to stay healthy. For example, Josie, who came for treatment to improve her fertility, now has treatment in order to stay well. When patients have preventative treatment they can continue to come for treatment every two to three months or at the change of season.

Preventative treatments can be compared to having a regular check-up with the dentist. A periodic visit to the dentist doesn't guarantee that you will not get a bad tooth between check-ups, but it can ensure that minor tooth problems are detected before they lead to major ones.

Ill-health often arises after major stresses or changes in your life. If you are having preventative treatment and further problems do arise you can always go back for more treatment when necessary. This can often help you to deal with such problems more effectively so that they don't cause major illnesses later on.

Treating degenerative conditions

A practitioner won't always be sure of how the patient will respond to treatment. If a patient has a chronic and degenerative condition such as multiple sclerosis, muscular dystrophy or Parkinson's disease their practitioner might tell them what she or he thinks treatment could achieve. Sometimes, although treatment may not give a complete cure, it can help a patient to feel more comfortable and to cope better with the complaint. How much can be accomplished in these situations is not always easy to assess until a few treatments have been carried out.

If your acupuncturist thinks that treatment will not help you, she or he will let you know or recommend another treatment that might be more beneficial. However, it is important to remember that your acupuncturist will ask 'Can acupuncture help this person?' rather than 'Can acupuncture help this illness?' One of the main differences between acupuncture and Western medicine is that the acupuncture practitioner treats people rather than diseases.

Summary

- Your acupuncturist will carry out a diagnosis during the first session. You may also receive a treatment although some practitioners prefer to wait until the next session. The first session can take up to one and a half hours.

- Treatments that are carried out at subsequent sessions take less time, lasting from half an hour to one hour.

- The needles have been pre-sterilised and the highest standards of hygiene are used when carrying out treatments.

- The needles are different from and very much finer than hypodermic needles.

- Patients do not describe the needles as painful. They describe a sensation that lasts for a few seconds, which can be an ache, numbness, a tingling or a sensation of heat.

- Four to ten needles are generally used per treatment although the number used depends on your condition.

- Besides needles your practitioner might use another treatment called moxibustion.

- Your practitioner will monitor your treatment to ensure it is working and will notice changes to your pulses and tongue as well as other areas such as your facial colour and the sparkle in your eyes.

- A patient with a chronic condition will usually begin having treatment once a week. Treatment will then be spread out as progress is made. Patients with acute conditions may initially need to come for treatment more frequently.

4

The Landscape of the Body: The Network of Qi Channels

When Craig had treatment for rheumatoid arthritis, some of the needles were used to unblock his pathways – or channels – of Qi. It was the obstruction in these pathways that had caused his severe joint pain and limited movement. In this chapter I will be describing these channels or pathways and the points that lie along them and I will also be discussing how they are used in treatment.

Samantha, who had a post-viral syndrome, also had blocked channels. Her pathways had become blocked by 'Dampness'. This made her feel extremely lethargic and heavy in her limbs as if she had a 'fat suit' on all of the time. The tiredness was so severe that even the smallest task was a terrible strain. Like Craig, she needed to have her channels unblocked and also to have the underlying Qi in her Organs supported and strengthened.

For Jenny and Josie the problem was different. Their complaints arose not from obstruction in the Qi pathways, but more directly from depletion of the Qi in their Organs. In Jenny's case her Heart function was treated in order to enable her to settle and overcome her nervousness and panic. In Josie's case her fertility problems were predominantly related to her Kidney function. Their treatment was still carried out by using points along the acupuncture channels but it focused on treating their Organs directly.

The 12 main channels

Your Qi and its circulation

So what is Qi circulation? You probably know you have blood circulating in your body but do you also know that there is another circulation system? The idea that there is a network of invisible pathways called 'channels' (sometimes known as 'meridians') spanning your whole body has been an integral part of the theory of Chinese medicine for thousands of years.

Qi – the energy flowing through the channels – is much less dense than matter, so you can't see it. It is nevertheless essential to your well-being. Qi is originally created from the combination of the air you breathe with the food you eat. This mixture then goes through several refining processes to become the Qi that moves through your channels. The Qi in your channels connects to and nourishes your Organs. I will discuss Qi in more detail in Chapter 6.

The channels and Organs

You can compare the channels and Organs to the landscape around you. If you had a bird's-eye view of most countries in the West, the first thing you'd probably notice are the roads. Some of these would be large dual carriageways where cars and lorries move from one major town to another. Other smaller roads give people access to more remote areas. The network of roads is similar to the network of channels that extend throughout your body.

The cities and towns can be compared to the Organs of the body. Often a road is named after the town it leads to. I come from Reading and in that town there is a Reading Road. In neighbouring Tilehurst is the Tilehurst Road. In the same way, the channels are named after the Organs they join up with.

Roads are vital links that bring supplies into the cities and towns. Sometimes roads become blocked. Most commonly nowadays this is due to traffic jams, but it can also be due to an accident, a fallen tree or even snowdrifts in winter. There might also be a food shortage, so that nothing is available to reach the cities or outposts. In both of these cases the residents become desperate when they don't have the provisions they need. If provisions are cut off for a long time, worse problems occur and looting and violence can even result.

Similarly, when the channels in the body become deficient or blocked, the organs are starved of vital Qi. If this continues for a long period, illness may arise in the body, mind or spirit. A problem affecting the Qi pathways alone is called a 'channel problem' in Chinese medicine.

Sometimes problems in urban areas are not due to poor road access but because there is unrest or pollution in the towns and cities themselves. The Organs of the body can be affected in much the same way. Rather than being weakened by lack of nourishment from the channels, they can be influenced directly by bad diet, pollution, injuries or emotional problems. In this case the cause of an illness is called an 'Organ problem'.

The connection between the channels and Organs

The 12 main channels and Organs are all connected. The Heart channel, which has pathways travelling down the arms, is joined to the Heart itself. The Small Intestine channel, which moves from the little finger across the shoulder blade and up to the face, has a branch that connects it to the Small Intestine Organ. Likewise the Stomach channel is connected to the Stomach Organ and the Gall Bladder channel to the Gall Bladder Organ.

Acupuncture often has an explanation for signs and symptoms that Western doctors puzzle over. This is because the diseases in question arise from imbalances in the channels and their connected Organs. Here are two examples. When patients are having heart problems, they often have a pain radiating down the arm to the little finger. The reason for this is hard for

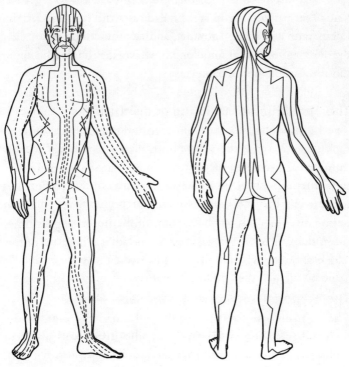

The channels

a Western medical doctor to understand, but it is easily explained by the fact that the acupuncture channel of the Heart travels down the little finger.

Another puzzle is why people who have headaches often feel nauseous at the same time. An acupuncturist understands that this is because many headaches are caused by an imbalance in the Gall Bladder. The Gall Bladder channel has numerous pathways travelling over the head and Gall Bladder problems can also lead to a feeling of nausea.

The 12 channels and Organs are paired together. Thus the Stomach is connected with the Spleen, the Gall Bladder with the Liver, and the Heart and Small Intestine are joined together. The other paired Organs are the Kidneys with the Bladder, the Lungs with the Large Intestine, and two functions, one called the Pericardium[1] and another known as the Triple Burner – more about these in Chapter 7.

The circulation of Qi in the main channels

The 12 main channels are connected and the Qi flows through each channel once every 24 hours, taking two hours to pass through each one. During this two-hour period your acupuncturist may choose to treat you on that channel to stoke up and support the Qi in the corresponding Organ. There is also a period of time (roughly 12 hours from the strongest time) when the Organ is at its weakest. Opposite is a diagram of this 'clock' showing when the Qi is at its two-hourly peak.

The complete network of channels

The 12 main pathways are not the only channels found in the body. The channel system forms a complete network that can be compared to the blood circulatory system with its network of blood vessels. The 12 main channels are similar to the

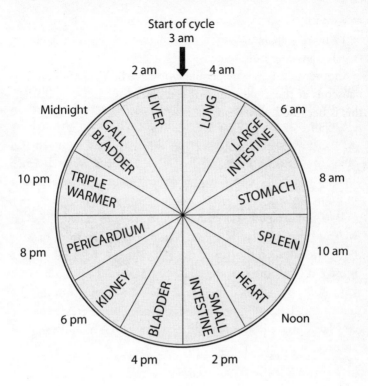

major blood vessels. These are connected to progressively smaller and smaller channels. The smallest channels are called 'cutaneous regions' and they lie on the surface of the body – rather like the capillaries that are the body's smallest blood vessels.

The different types of channels are as follows, in order of their size:

- 12 primary/main channels
- 8 extraordinary channels
- 12 divergent channels

- 15 connecting channels
- 12 muscle channels
- 12 cutaneous regions

Some of these channels are very important to an acupuncturist, most notably the Extraordinary Channels. These eight channels help to regulate the Qi in your 12 main channels by acting as reservoirs and ensuring that you have sufficient Qi circulating in your body. They also circulate your Essence around the body (see Chapter 6) and help to regulate your immune system.

Two important Extraordinary Channels are called the Ren Mai and the Du Mai. The Ren Mai travels up the front of your body and is called the 'sea of the Yin channels' because it is the most Yin of all the channels. The Du Mai runs up the back of your body and is called the 'sea of the Yang channels' as it is the most Yang. Treatment on these two channels can create balance and harmony within your Yin and Yang Qi. Yin and Yang are covered in detail in Chapter 6.

The acupuncture points

What is an acupuncture point?

Most of the body's acupuncture points lie along each of the 12 main channels, along with the Ren Mai and Du Mai. Points are best imagined as small whirlpools or vortices that are formed where the flow of Qi is disrupted. They are often found at prominences or indentations along the pathways such as where a bone flares at a joint, where there is a notch in a bone or where two muscles meet. This is similar to the way small whirlpools are formed when the smooth flow of a stream or river is disrupted.

The acupuncture points are used in treatment to either strengthen or unblock the Qi in the channels. By stimulating the points with a needle the flow of the Qi is altered. The Qi can then reach a better balance and flow unimpeded to the Organs, allowing their functioning to improve. Hence you can regain your health.

The number of points on the body

There are approximately 365 points on the body and each has an individual use. Sometimes the points are used in combination to create a more powerful effect and at other times points are chosen individually.

Some channels have more points on them than others. There are 67 points on the Bladder channel, for instance, while there are only nine each on the Pericardium and Heart pathways. Points are identified by their name and also by their associated Organ and a number. For example, the point in the box below is called 'Stomach 36' because it is the 36th point along the Stomach channel.

Stomach 36 – the 'chicken soup point' of the body

Stomach 36 can be compared to chicken soup – one of the most nourishing dishes in Chinese cuisine. This is because it is one of the most powerful points on the body. It lies on the Stomach channel and is located on the lower leg. All points have their own names and this one is called 'Leg Three Miles'. It is often used to strengthen a patient with depleted energy: after using it, it is said that the patient will be able to walk another three miles! This point has many other functions and can benefit a patient's body, mind and spirit. For example, physically it has a strong effect on the digestive system and the stomach. It can also influence the immune system, having the ability to strengthen resistance to infections. It can bring great stability to people who are feeling emotionally unstable or insecure. It helps to calm the mind and spirit of those who are worried, anxious or obsessive. It can also clear the mind if a patient has been studying intensively or over-thinking.

Different types of points

The points on the 12 main channels have many different uses, of which some are more physical and others have more effect on the mind and spirit.

Certain other points on the body are called 'extraordinary' points. These are important points but they don't lie on the 12 main channels. For example, the name of one extra-ordinary point on the neck is translated 'Peaceful Sleep' because of its relaxing effects, and there are also two points by the knee that are called 'The Eyes of the Knee'. The Eyes of the Knee give impressive results in the treatment of many knee problems.

Although acupuncture is 2,000 years old, new points are sometimes discovered and these can prove extremely useful. For example, there is a point just below Stomach 36 on the Stomach channel that becomes tender on pressure if a patient's appendix is inflamed. Knowing about this point can help to clarify the the diagnosis of appendicitis when a patient has abdominal pain.

Some other points can also become tender with pressure. One famous Chinese doctor called Sun Si Miao (pronounced 'Sun See Me-ow') is reputed to have said: 'If an area is tender then it is an acupuncture point.' Places which feel tender on pressure, especially those around joints or painful areas, are called *ah shi* points in Chinese (pronounced 'ar sher'). *Ah shi* is translated as 'Oh yes'. When the practitioner presses the right spot the patient says, 'Oh yes, that's where it is!'

Finding the points

Not all acupuncture points are found by sensitivity to pressure but all of their locations can be accurately found by locating specified landmarks on the body. For example, the first point on the Gall Bladder channel is located next to the outer corner of the eye and the last point on the Bladder channel is next to the nail point of the little toe. Students spend many years learning to locate each of these points and in the process cultivate a very refined and sensitive sense of touch.

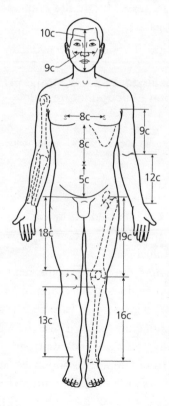

Cun **measurements**

Chinese medical doctors also invented a clever method of finding points by measurement. Using this method the practitioner divides an area of the body into equal parts. For example, the forearm is divided into 12 equal portions known as *cun* (pronounced 'sun'). The Pericardium is a channel that runs up the centre of the forearm. One point on this channel lies at two *cun* from the wrist crease, another is at three, while yet another lies five *cun* away. By using this method of measurement the points can all be found accurately and an acupuncturist can always locate the points no matter what a person's size or shape.

Ancient Chinese doctors – *Wang Wei Yi* and the standardisation of acupuncture points

The locations for all acupuncture points were first standardised by a famous Chinese doctor called *Wang Wei Yi* (pronounced 'Wong Way Ye'), in AD 1026. He wrote a book called *Tongren shuxue zhenjui*

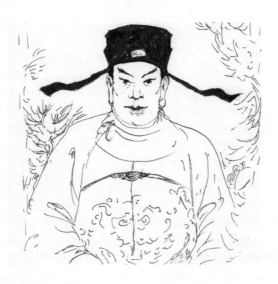

tujing – The Illustrated Manual for Acupuncture and Moxibustion – which was published by the Imperial Court. The Emperor then commissioned two 'bronze men' to be cast showing the locations of the acupuncture points. *Wang Wei Yi* oversaw the process to make sure that it was accurately carried out. These first bronze figures were kept in the Emperor's palace. More bronze figures were subsequently made. The acupuncture points on the figure were made by punching tiny holes through the bronze. During students' examinations the bronze man was covered in wax and filled with water. If the student located the acupuncture points correctly the needle went through the wax, water would pour from the holes and the student had passed the exam!

Choosing where to place the needles

When your acupuncturist decides where to place the needles, she or he will first decide on 'treatment principles' based on the diagnosis. The points to use will then be chosen based on these principles. For example, Josie had a constitutional imbalance in her Bladder and Kidney function and much of her treatment was centred on strengthening those Organs. When she was treated for infertility she also had treatment to warm her lower abdomen. Directly after her mother died, much of her treatment was directed at giving her emotional support. Through the course of all of this treatment the main treatment principles I used were designed to strengthen her Bladder and Kidney function, warm her lower abdomen and calm her mind and spirit.

Having decided on treatment principles, the practitioner will decide on the particular points to use. Most of the points are on the arms or legs, although points on other areas of the body such as the back, chest or abdomen may be used. These will be chosen for three main reasons:

- They lie on channels connected with the Organs which are imbalanced (see Chapter 7 for more on this)
- They have special functions that will enhance the treatment
- The name of the point indicates that the use of that point is appropriate.

Because Josie needed treatment on her Bladder and Kidney channels many of the points I used for her treatment were along these channels. A point on her lower abdomen that was beneficial was called 'Door of Infants' – the name of this point in relation to its use for fertility problems speaks for itself. An example of a point used to calm her mind and spirit was a point on her Heart channel at her wrist. This is called 'Spirit Gate' and it has a particularly calming action.

Heart 7 – The Spirit Gate

This is one of the most frequently used points on the Heart channel. It is a very flexible point with a wide variety of uses. Its name, 'Spirit Gate', may give us some insight into its ability to strongly affect the spirit of the Heart. Spirit Gate was also a name given by many Daoists to the eyes[2] and it is via the eyes that the practitioner can notice the vitality and brightness of a person's spirit. This point is an excellent one to use when a patient is feeling unsettled or agitated and it will often have an immediate calming effect during the treatment. It lies on the wrist and although it is located at a great distance from the Heart it can physically strengthen this Organ when a patient has physical heart problems.

Josie described the effect of this point, telling me, 'Whenever I had one particular point on my wrist treated I would feel a whoosh of energy travelling straight up the inside of my arm, over my head and down my other arm. I then felt completely at peace and didn't want to move.' She had experienced the energy of the Heart channel moving through its pathway and the resulting well-being and relaxation.

Are the same points used at every treatment?

Sometimes acupuncturists will use the same points for a number of treatments and at other times they will need to change the point more frequently. This depends on each patient and the nature of their condition. Josie's and Jenny's points were changed quite frequently. This was because as they were progressing and changing internally, their needs were shifting. A point which benefited them one week was often no longer appropriate at the next visit.

Craig, on the other hand, often had the same points treated. This was because his channels were blocked and treatment gradually cleared the blockage. Some of the same points were used at every treatment for a while.

Restoring your health

Imbalances in the channels or Organs are produced by emotional, climatic or lifestyle causes of disease. By understanding these causes, patients may be encouraged to change their lifestyle when it is necessary. This, in turn, can help treatment to progress more rapidly and prevent a recurrence of an illness. I will be discussing some of these causes of disease in the next two chapters.

Summary

- There are 12 main channels on the body and each is connected to and named after one of six Yin and six Yang Organs.
- Qi flows through each of the 12 main channels once every 24 hours, taking two hours to pass through each one. This is often called the 'Chinese clock'.

- The complete system of Qi circulation can be compared to the circulation of blood in the body, with large channels and smaller cutaneous channels on the surface of the body.
- The body's acupuncture points lie along the channels. They are often found at prominences or indentations along the pathways. They are used in treatment either to strengthen or unblock the Qi in the channels.
- A practitioner will choose points for three main reasons:
  - Because they are located on channels connected with the Organs which are imbalanced
  - Because they have special functions that will enhance the treatment
  - Because the name of the point indicates that the use of that point is appropriate.

5

Why Do We Get Ill?
Our External and Internal
Climate

Why we become ill

The importance of 'old wives' tales'

When I was young my mother would often say things like, 'Don't sleep in a draught, you'll get a stiff neck' or 'Don't go out with wet hair, you'll catch a chill.' At other times she would tell me, 'Don't sit on hot radiators' or 'Put your slippers on, dear' or when I'd played happily in the rain, 'Change out of those damp clothes, dear.' All of these warnings fell on deaf ears, and I definitely forgot about them when I became an adult and didn't have to do as I was told any more. Then I learned Chinese medicine . . .

When I studied Chinese medicine I discovered the importance of these 'old wives' tales'. They now became 'golden rules'.

I busily started telling my patients about them so that they too could learn to look after themselves and be protected against the elements of Cold, Damp, Wind, Heat and Dryness. There were also some other sayings that I realised I could have taken more seriously when I was younger. Some were about my lifestyle, such as, 'It's important to have at least one hot meal a day' or 'The hours of sleep before midnight are twice as good as those after' or 'All work and no play makes Jack/Jill a dull boy/girl.' Other sayings were about how we look after ourselves emotionally. The Chinese are very strong on these and have proverbs like 'Laugh three times a day to live longer' and 'A soft temper is the root of a long life.'

Some examples of well-known 'old wives' tales'

- Don't sit on wet grass.
- Don't sit on stone steps.
- Change out of wet clothes.
- Don't sleep with your head facing a fire or radiator.
- Dry your washed hair before going out.
- Don't swim or wash your hair during your period.
- Always wear a hat when it's cold.
- Don't go to sleep with wet hair.
- Cover your neck in the wind.
- Avoid sitting or sleeping in a draught.
- Air your clothes before wearing them.
- Don't sit in the midday sun.
- Don't walk on cold floors without shoes on.
- Add or take off extra clothes when you change from a warm to a cold environment.
- Don't leave your back or abdomen uncovered.
- Don't make love during a period.
- When travelling home from abroad wrap up warmly for when the temperature drops.
- Don't sit on hot radiators.
- Dry yourself thoroughly after bathing.
- Don't swim when you have a cold.
- Wear a vest.

The 'golden rules' – East and West

Over time I realised that all cultures had certain 'health rules' which were passed down from generation to generation and which many people adhered to. Even in the West until the late nineteenth century, ill-health was regarded as a lack of harmony between a sick person and their environment.[1] It is from this philosophy that such 'old wives' tales' arose. With the coming of modern technology and modern ways of thinking, however, this understanding was lost in the Western world. Chinese medicine, however, didn't forget the essence of these guidelines, and in this chapter you will learn more about them and what you can do to remain healthy.

The multiple causes of disease

Everybody has their own set of very individual circumstances that may lead to them becoming ill. In Chapter 2 you read the stories of acupuncture patients who talked about their treatment and gave reasons why they became unwell. You may have noticed that they often gave more than one reason. For example, Samantha, Jenny, Francesca and Josie cited different emotional stresses including a marriage break-up, panic over university coursework, a stressful job and the death of a parent as contributing to their illnesses. Running alongside, however, they knew that there were other factors such as poor diet, the cold and damp weather, a bad car accident or too much exercise. Sarah noticed that emotional issues played a part in her illness although her specific problem arose after a chest infection.

How important is it to know what caused my problem?

There is no need for you to know the cause of your illness in order to become healthy again. Craig's arthritis responded to treatment very quickly and he never really knew why it came on. Sometimes, however, it can be helpful to know what the cause is.

The more you know about why illnesses arise, the more you can do to prevent them. For instance, if you know that you get headaches when you are tense at work, you might think twice about getting involved in stressful situations that could bring them on. If you know you are susceptible to feeling cold, or dislike windy weather, then you might wrap up well in that kind of climate.

The motivation to stay healthy has been deeply ingrained in Chinese culture for thousands of years. From generation to generation people have studied how their health is affected by their lifestyle and this knowledge has been passed on through succeeding generations. The census held in the UK in 1991 illustrated the benefits this has on the health of Chinese people. The census found that only 29 per cent of Chinese pensioners had long-lasting illnesses compared to 36 per cent of white people and 43 per cent of people of Indian or Pakistani origin.[2] These results are especially stunning because the Chinese people included in this census were living in an unfamiliar culture. In the West, many people now have a much greater understanding of the need to stay healthy and we have much to learn from Chinese medicine.

The major causes of disease

The Chinese medicine understood that there are three general areas from which disease arises. They called these the external, the internal and the miscellaneous causes of disease.[3]

The external causes of disease are climatic conditions – the kind of things I was warned about in 'old wives' tales'. The internal causes of disease come from inside you and are to do with your emotions. The miscellaneous causes of disease are sometimes referred to as 'lifestyle' causes. They include factors such as diet, exercise, work and rest.

I've divided the rest of this chapter into three parts. In each part I'll cover one of these areas, starting with the external ones.

The external causes of disease

The external causes of disease come from climatic conditions. These pathogens are called Cold, Damp, Wind, Heat and Dryness.

Cold

The Chinese described Cold as something that stops movement and warmth and makes people's tissues contract. Pain results from this contraction. A friend's description of wintry weather explains this well: 'I used to feel the cold badly when I was young and I hated it. It wasn't so much feeling chilly that got to me, it was more the awful pain in my hands and feet that I disliked. I sometimes even felt it in my ears or my nose'.

Chinese medicine teaches that cold contracts the body and, in the case of my friend, her peripheral circulation. It may surprise you to know that in spite of improved housing and warm clothes, the cold is responsible for more deaths and other health disorders than most other weather conditions. The elderly, young and frail are most affected but we are all susceptible and many illnesses are due to the cold.

There are more strokes, heart attacks and respiratory infections in the winter. The winter of 1963 was one of the coldest in France since the beginning of the century. In that year the mortality of people over 60 years old increased by 15.7 per cent compared to the previous winter.[4] Chilblains are one of the most obvious results of extreme cold. They are caused by a narrowing of the blood vessels just below the skin. Cold can also affect the tendons, causing your joints to become painful, white and contracted.

Am I susceptible to Cold?

1. Do you dislike being out in cold weather?
2. Do you want to turn on the electric blanket or have a hot water bottle as soon as the temperature drops even slightly?
3. If you are out in the cold do you urinate more?
4. Do you crave holidays in sunny climates?

If the answer to at least two of these questions is Yes, you may be susceptible to Cold.

Chronic diarrhoea, stomach pains or an inability to digest food can also result from eating too much cold food, as can period pains or no periods at all. Another frequent cause of bowel or period problems is Cold caught in the lower abdomen. An acupuncturist can clear Cold from a person's system by using moxibustion alongside needles. This may be used on a specific area such as the stomach, lower abdomen or lower back, or used more generally to warm a person who easily feels the cold.

The following are some ways in which you can protect yourself from the effects of Cold:

- Wear many layers of clothes to trap the heat.
- Take notice of sharp pains when you are out in the cold – pain in the ears, hands, feet or head can be a warning to cover up.
- Avoid sitting on stone or metal seats without insulation.
- Avoid cold foods such as iced drinks or food taken straight from the fridge.
- Keep your environment adequately heated.
- Keep your torso covered (despite the fact that it's fashionable to have it uncovered) to avoid Cold 'invading' the abdomen.

Damp

Damp is a very common cause of problems for many people in the UK and other countries that are wet or humid. When I teach UK students about Damp, everyone believes that where they come from is the dampest area in Britain!

People don't have to live in a damp area to be injured by Damp. Living in a damp house, staying by or on water, remaining in wet clothes or even doing what the old wives warned you about – sitting on damp grass – can all affect people if they are vulnerable.

If you feel heavy-limbed, ache, are lethargic and a bit depressed on a damp or humid day you have already experienced some of the effects of Damp. Damp can also make people feel so heavy that they want to lie down. A patient with symptoms of Damp told me that her favourite saying was, 'Why stand when you can sit, and why sit when you can lie down?'

Am I susceptible to retaining Damp?

1. Do you feel worse in damp weather?
2. Do you easily bloat up in your abdomen or stomach?
3. Do you sometimes feel heavy in your limbs or head?
4. Do you often want to lie down?
5. Do you sometimes feel muzzy-headed or lack concentration?

If the answer to three or more of these questions is Yes then you may be susceptible to Damp.

Some other symptoms of Damp are feeling stuffy in the chest, bloated in the stomach or abdomen, heavy in the head and lacking in concentration or energy. In the lower part of the body this pathogen can cause bowel problems, fluid retention, discharges or a heavy feeling in the legs. Samantha, who talked about her treatment for post-viral syndrome in Chapter 2, described some symptoms of Damp when she told me, 'There was no tiredness like it. It was like my blood had been replaced with lead and like I had a big fat suit on all the time with heavy weights hanging from it.'

An acupuncturist will often use points on the Spleen channel to clear Damp. This patient describes how she felt when she had Damp cleared: 'At one treatment the needles were put in at the sides of my knees. I felt as if something was flushed out of my body in a gush. I came out of treatment with a spring in my step.'

Some people are more susceptible to Damp than others. Unlike Wind (see below), which comes and goes quickly, Damp is said to be 'sticky and lingering' and is difficult to clear.

The following are some ways in which you can protect yourself from the effects of Damp:

- Make sure you keep your environment dry – buy a de-humidifier to dry out a damp house.
- Keep your body dry – dry yourself thoroughly after bathing.
- Don't sleep with wet hair and don't sit around in damp places.
- Wear dry clothes – air them thoroughly and change out of clothes that get wet.
- If your clothes get damp from sweating, change out of them once you have finished sweating – waiting until you have finished allows your pores to close first.
- If you are susceptible to Damp cut down on sticky 'Damp-forming' foods such as dairy produce, greasy foods, and wheat.

Wind

One of my patients recently had a cold. This is a good example of what Chinese medicine calls an invasion of Wind-Cold: 'I felt fine the day before. In the middle of the night I woke up with a sore throat and knew I was in for an infection. The next day I felt terrible. My nose was running, my jaw ached, my eyes hurt, and I felt extremely tired and shivery. Two days later all my symptoms had gone during the day, yet I still woke up coughing at night. It was five days before it went completely.'

What the Chinese call Wind in the body closely matches what they observe in the environment. Wind is something that arises suddenly and goes through many rapid changes. It is often located on the outside of the body and moves in an upward direction. My patient's cold had all of these qualities. She also felt very shivery with her cold as Cold was mixed with the Wind affecting her body.

Am I susceptible to Wind?

1. Are you easily affected by changes in temperature, windy weather or draughts?

2. Do you ever have pains that move position or come and go?
3. Do you ever have itchy skin, painful ears, eyes or nose, sneezing or shivering when exposed to draughts or changes in temperature?
4. Do you catch colds easily?

If the answer to at least two of these questions is Yes, you may be easily affected by Wind.

Other symptoms that Chinese medicine describes as arising from Wind are joint pains that move from place to place, symptoms that come and go (such as skin problems or twitches), and symptoms that make us shake or move, such as epilepsy or strokes.

There are two main ways in which people can be affected by Wind. The first is by being caught in 'windy' conditions. These can include a windy day, a draught, a breeze from a fan or even air conditioning. The second situation described as 'Wind' is a sudden weather change such as unseasonable weather conditions, moving in and out of shops and other heated environments, or returning from holidays abroad.

Research carried out as far back as the late 1950s provided some understanding of the effects of wind or changes in the weather on our health. Researchers were able to establish that many rheumatic attacks that were severe enough for a person to stop work were often related to changes in the weather. They found that the most harmful meteorological events are a sudden drop in temperature, strong winds and the influx of polar air masses.[5]

Often patients don't know exactly why they have 'caught' or, as Chinese medicine would say, are 'invaded' by Wind and Cold, but this doesn't matter. To have the symptoms of Wind is enough to make a diagnosis. Having said that, severe windy weather affecting our health has been well documented in many countries. If the patient described above had taken more notice of the old wives' tales, however, she might have taken better care of herself and avoided getting ill.

Acupuncture treatment can be used specifically to clear Wind from your body. For instance, many acupuncture points have the word 'Wind' in their name: 'Wind Pond', 'Wind Gate' and 'Wind Palace' are a few examples. Using these and other points will help to clear this condition.

The following are some ways in which you can protect yourself from the effects of Wind:

- Wrap up against windy or cold weather.
- Don't sit or sleep in a draught or in front of a fan.
- Beware of changes in temperature – such as moving from a warm environment to a cooler outside temperature.
- Keep your neck and head covered in windy weather.
- Don't go out with wet hair or sleep without drying your hair.
- Don't exercise in the wind.

Heat

I love the sun. After a long hard winter there's nothing more likely to get me out of the house and socialising. In general people are better equipped to deal with Heat than Cold. Heat is very comforting and soothing when you're feeling chilly. Heat can also be destructive, however. If you are already hot it can make you extremely restless and be very distracting. When Heat disturbs people it moves upwards to their heads and can make them irritable – 'hot-headed' is an apt term used for people who are hot and bothered and angry.

Am I susceptible to Heat?

1. Do you get uncomfortably hot in warm weather?
2. Do you ever wake even on a cool-ish night wanting to remove some of the bedcovers?
3. Do you tend to get restless when a room is too hot?
4. Do you find you need to wear fewer clothes than many of your friends?

If the answer to two or more of these questions is Yes then you may be susceptible to Heat.

Sunstroke is the most obvious example of how people might be affected by external Heat. People who work in a laundry or a hot kitchen may also be prone to suffer Heat conditions, as will people who already have a slight tendency to feel hot. Heat can show itself in one area only, such as a red, hot, painful joint. It may also be all over the body in the form of hot flushes. Heat can also combine with Damp causing infectious or very inflamed conditions that are both hot and full of pus. When you have an infection with a high fever, Chinese medicine would say you are affected by a combination of Wind and Heat.

Sometimes Wind, Damp or Cold, trapped in the body for a long time, can start generating Heat. One good example of this is cold, painful joints suddenly becoming inflamed and extremely hot.

An acupuncturist will deal with excessive Heat in two main ways. One way is to treat specific points that are used to clear Heat. The other way is to 'put the fire out' by using points that bring moisture and coolness to the body.

The following are some ways in which you can protect yourself from the effects of Heat:

- Don't stay out in the sun for very long periods – especially avoid the midday sun.
- Build up slowly to acclimatise yourself to the sun or very hot environments.
- Drink lots of fluids to avoid dehydrating.
- Protect your skin with sun creams.
- Wear clothes to protect yourself – tops with sleeves to protect the arms, and hats to protect the head and face.
- If susceptible to heat, avoid 'heating' foods such as curries, and meats such as lamb or beef.

Dryness

When I went on my first trip to China, one of my friends on the trip became ill. She describes her symptoms as follows: 'I remember stepping outside in Beijing and breathing in. I had the extraordinary feeling of the cold and dryness going through my nose and deep into my lungs. A few days later it turned into an infection. It was unlike anything I'd experienced before. I had a feeling of incredible dryness in my lungs and an aching feeling in my chest. I had a hacking cough but no matter how much I coughed I just couldn't produce anything.'

She was experiencing an 'attack' of Dryness. For most of you, symptoms of Dryness are likely to come either from central heating or during aeroplane flights.

Am I susceptible to Dryness?

1. Do you get thirsty easily?
2. Do you have a tendency to get dry skin?
3. Do you quite enjoy damp weather but hate dryness?

4. Do you easily get a dry cough?

If the answer to at least two of these questions is Yes then you may have a tendency towards dryness.

Dryness is extremely rare in the UK as it is such a damp country. Dryness can create any 'dry' symptoms but will often cause a dry nose, throat, lungs or dry skin. Points on the Lung channel are often used to clear it.

The following are some ways in which you can protect yourself from the effects of Dryness:

- Place a small bowl of water in a room to ease a dry atmosphere, especially if it is caused by central heating.
- If you are in a really dry environment, buy a humidifier.
- Breathe in steam from a bowl of hot water or use a vaporiser if you're suffering from a dry cough.
- Drink lots of water in the drying atmosphere of a plane to avoid dehydration.

How do climatic influences affect the body?

Under normal circumstances most people can 'brave the elements' with ease and will not be adversely affected by them. There are two common situations when these pathogens can have a detrimental effect. The first is when you are already weakened or susceptible to climatic conditions and the second is if the climatic influence is so extreme that you can't resist it.

If you feel the cold easily you will be more susceptible to Cold conditions, whereas if you are of a hotter constitution you will be more easily affected by Heat. People who are affected by damp weather often have weakened Spleen energy (more about this in Chapter 7).

Sub-zero temperatures, a tropical climate or severely humid weather can take their toll on even the healthiest people. One of my patients who originated from near Newcastle describes how the elements affected her as a child: 'I had rheumatism every winter from the age of 7 to 16 years. I couldn't pick up a pen to write or play with my friends as I could hardly walk. I lived on the north-east coast of England where the winds were vicious, cold and damp. At the age of 16 I spent three weeks in the Alps where we had solid hot, dry sunshine. I suppose it dried me out. That was the first winter that I didn't have rheumatism. After that I moved to the south of England and didn't go back to the north-east. I never had it again.'

This patient was lucky. The climatic condition that affected her was 'dried out' naturally by the sun. When a condition won't clear by itself acupuncture can then be very helpful.

The internal causes of disease

Even as far back as 2,000 years ago Chinese medicine understood that people's emotional states are major factors in their ability to remain healthy. Thankfully, this link between our emotions and our health is now being increasingly accepted and backed up by scientific studies. For example, one study beginning in the 1940s found that people who are optimistic are likely to be healthier later on in their life than those who are pessimistic. In this study 99 healthy and successful graduates from Harvard University filled out questionnaires that determined their level of optimism or pessimism. They then completed questionnaires each year and were examined by a physician every five years until the age of 60. Although all graduates were healthy when they left Harvard, the results showed that pessimism in early adulthood is a risk factor for ill-health in middle and late adulthood. By the age of 60, 13 of these people had died. Those who were more optimistic remained in better health and were at their healthiest between 40 and 45. Stunningly, there was a less than 1 in 1,000 chance that these results were random – not even the statistical link between lung cancer and smoking is as strong as that![6]

If laughter and optimism have positive effects on our health, what are the effects of negative emotions?

The internal 'climate'

Just as there is an external climate, so our emotions can be likened to an internal 'climate'. The internal causes of disease are anger, grief, fear, shock, worry, over-thinking and joy. Although Chinese medicine named only these seven emotions as causes of disease, they include all other emotions. For example, anger can include frustration, depression, resentment, irritation, bitterness and rage. Fear can also encompass fright, terror, dread or anxiety. Grief can include emptiness, longing, regret or remorse.

How emotions can affect you

It is normal and healthy for people to express emotions in certain situations. For example, you will naturally feel afraid if you are physically threatened and you will normally feel angry if you are badly let down. When the situation has been rectified, for example if the threat is removed or the person who let you down has apologised, then you can move on in life rather than becoming stuck in these feelings.

Sometimes emotions are not so easily resolved. They may be prolonged or intense or it may be that they are never expressed properly or acknowledged. In this case they can become a cause of disease.

How emotions can make us ill

The roots of an internal cause of disease are often established at a very early age. People have no control over their emotions when they are babies and they howl with rage if frustrated, feel frightened if threatened, or feel sad if left for an overly long period. Their emotional state changes rapidly. In time, most people pass through these feelings and move on to other states as their circumstances alter.

Common stresses at different stages of our lives[7]

Childhood 0–5
Lack of food; lack of warm environment; lack of emotional warmth and stimulation; lack of ability to get emotional needs met; lack of or too many physical boundaries; sibling rivalries; difficulty in separating from parents as grow older.

Childhood 5–12
Starting school; making friends; learning difficulties; sibling rivalries; bullying; moving home; parents divorcing; keeping up with schoolwork; too much television or computer work.

Teenage years 13–19
Starting relationships with same or opposite sex; making friends; concern about appearance; fear of failing exams; difficulties choosing a career; becoming independent from parents; experimenting with drugs and/or alcohol; finding work; leaving home.

Adulthood 20–40
Finding a partner; building a home; starting a family; finding and settling in a career; financial worries and debts; competitive work situation; difficult boss; difficulties with colleagues; relationship problems; divorce.

Late adulthood 40–60

Redundancies; lack of promotion; keeping up with changes in technology at work; caring for ageing parents; family illness; death of relatives and friends; advancing age; poorer health; divorce.

Retirement 60+

Lack of feeling valued; death of loved ones; failing health; advancing age; failing eyesight, hearing, memory, etc.; loss of income; loss of ability to care for oneself; difficulty maintaining independence.

Over time, however, if people frequently have the experience of feeling frustrated, frightened or sad, chronic emotional patterns develop which may weaken their Qi. These patterns evolve into repetitive emotional states in adult life.

Some people have difficulty in expressing their anger, others easily feel anxious and frightened, yet others worry incessantly or often feel joyless and sad for no good reason. To understand these emotions better I'll look at each of them in turn so that you can find out more about how they can influence your health.

Anger

The Chinese say that anger most often affects the Liver. Anger can be anything from resentment, irritability and frustration to extreme rage. It can also lead to depression when it is not expressed.

Anger is most often seen as a negative emotion. It can be very destructive if it is uncontrolled, causing physical fights, rows and ultimately relationship breakdowns. At the other extreme, anger can be a very positive emotion, leading people to fight for justice or stand up for themselves and others if they have been abused or let down. Short-term anger or frustration that has a resolution is healthy. More enduring unresolved feelings that cause long-term anger and resentment, on the other hand, can lead to ill-health.

Anger and its effect on your health

The Chinese say that anger makes Qi rise[8] and in Chinese medicine it is often associated with headaches. Research at the St Louis University School of Medicine in the USA confirms this connection. In one study 171 people with chronic headaches were compared with a similar number who were headache free. It was found that those with headaches were much more likely to hold their anger in than those who did not get headaches. Conversely, the study also found that when anger was not expressed it became more likely that a person would succumb to a headache.[9]

A study carried out in Japan on 4,374 people with high blood pressure concluded that those who do not express anger have an increased risk of high blood pressure.[10] For a long time people have been urged to relax to reduce high blood pressure but research suggests that finding ways to deal with their anger is more important. Your acupuncturist will agree. High blood pressure is often associated with unresolved feelings of anger and the functioning of the Liver.

Not everyone holds their anger in. Others find they are letting it out too readily. This can also affect people's health in a negative way. In consumer research carried out by National Opinion Polls, it was found that 90 per cent of people said they now flare up more than they did ten years ago and 10 per cent of people said they lose their temper more than once a day. Being kept on hold on the phone was considered the most stressful situation, closely followed by frustrations in traffic causing road rage.[11]

Ancient Chinese doctors – *Hua Tuo* and his cure using anger

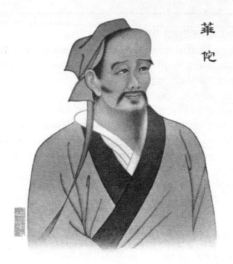

Hua Tuo (pronounced 'Hwa Toe') was born in AD 120. He started life as a woodcutter and later practised many different Chinese medical treatments. *Hua Tuo* was noted for his ability to transmit his own energy through acupuncture needles and for his simple yet beneficial remedies. He was said to have cured a certain General *Cao Cao* of his chronic headaches with only one acupuncture treatment.

A legendary story about *Hua Tuo* tells of his clever and courageous treatment of a high-ranking official. When *Hua Tuo* examined his patient he became aware that the official needed to become angry and that this was the only cure for his serious illness. *Hua Tuo* took a large consultation fee and disappeared leaving an insolent letter. The official sent his guards to capture *Hua Tuo*, who went into hiding. When the guards were unable to find him the official was so angry that he vomited and was instantly restored to health.

Grief

Grief is another emotion that can have a strong effect on our health. It can be described as sorrow, regret, sadness, a sense of remorse or a sense of loss. Grief affects the Lungs and people weep when they release their grief.

Grief is expressed differently in different cultures. In the UK many people keep a 'stiff upper lip' and often find it difficult to express their true feelings when someone dies or goes away. In contrast, in the East a 'celebration of the white' is held. This is a funeral party where white is worn (white being the colour associated with the Lungs and grief) as an outward manifestation of the grieving process. Wreaths are placed outside the entrance of the home and over a three-day period, which is the established time for the passing of the dead, the guests eat, drink, play mah-jong and talk.[12] Chinese medicine teaches that if grief is expressed there is less chance of illness arising than if it is held inside.

Grief and its effect on your health

Research has confirmed that grief following bereavement often results in an increased risk of illness. One study held at the University of Aarhus in Denmark found that there was an increased risk of a heart attack in bereaved parents. This is not surprising, as the death of a child is probably one of the most difficult losses that can be experienced. It was found that the risk was highest in those who suffered the loss unexpectedly, for example in cases of sudden infant death syndrome.[13]

The effects of an unexpressed loss can often be helped by acupuncture treatment. One of my patients told me, 'After my first treatment I cried for the whole day. I realised it was the grief I didn't express when my mother died. I then felt much better.'

Grief takes many forms. Some people feel a loss, not because someone has died or gone away but because they haven't achieved what they wanted to in life – what they have lost is a dream but they may still feel just as bereft. Any loss can be devastating and a cause of illness.

Fear and shock

Fear and fright affect the Kidneys. Fright can also affect the Heart. Fear or fright can be devastating and many people feel it constantly. Josie, who first came to be treated for infertility, also suffered from many fears before finding acupuncture. She told me, 'When I first came for treatment my mind would run away with me and I'd imagine all sorts of things happening to my husband. It got worse before my period and sometimes stopped me sleeping at night.'

Following treatment using points on her Bladder and Kidneys, her fear lessened and she said, 'Things don't bother me now as they did. I feel much calmer and more peaceful inside. I'm also more independent and don't worry if my husband is out of the house.'

Fear and its effect on your health

Fear can be a positive way to help us to be cautious. At the other extreme, it can also disable us because of imagined catastrophes. A study carried out at the Stanford School of Medicine in the USA found that of women who had had heart attacks, the ones who went on to have a second one were those who were the most fearful. In many cases these were women who had chronic fears and who may have stopped driving, left their job or stopped going out.[14]

Here is how one of my patients described what happens when he gets frightened: 'When I'm frightened, I breathe more rapidly. My stomach feels tense and I can't concentrate. I can be lying in the bath relaxing and reading and see the dark passage out of the corner of my eye and that sets me off. Once a light bulb blew when I put it in, and it brought on a panic attack.'

At the other end of the spectrum are situations where people feel no fear although they are in danger. Evel Knievel was an example of someone who loved to perform daredevil stunts. When he finally retired in 1981 he'd broken 35 bones, been operated on 15 times and spent three years of his life in hospital, but shrugged it off as 'the price you pay for success'! Most examples of feeling no fear are of course not so extreme: for instance, many people drive too fast. Fear and the lack of it can both cause later ill-health. When we are afraid or do something dangerous, adrenalin is pumped around the body and the resulting tension strains our organs.

The inner smile

This well-known Chinese exercise takes only a few minutes to do. It relaxes and rejuvenates the internal organs and helps us through any tense situation. We can do this exercise at any time – sitting in the office, in a stressful meeting or when studying for exams. It will make any difficulties easier to cope with.

Sit with your back straight.

Imagine seeing something that will make you smile. Allow yourself to smile internally – it doesn't have to be visible, only felt by you.

Allow the smile to shine out of your eyes.

Now let the smile travel downwards into all of your internal organs. Notice the feeling of relaxation generated by the internal smile.

Allow the smile to travel down to your *dan tian*, an important energy centre just below the navel which is the root of our physical energy.

Carry on with what you are doing, keeping the feeling generated by the internal smile. Others will also respond to the good feelings activated by your internal smile.

Worry and over-thinking

Two other common states that put a strain on your health are worry and over-thinking. Although over-thinking is not strictly speaking an emotion, it is still an internal cause of disease. Worry and over-thinking affect people's Spleen and Stomach Qi and can include too much studying, obsessive thinking or continually working over something in your mind.

Worry can gnaw away at some people, even when there is nothing to be concerned about. Here, one of my patients tells me about how she was affected by obsessive thoughts: 'I got worked up when I got a pain in my breast. The doctor reassured me but I kept thinking it was cancer. I started to feel sick and I'd keep thinking of a friend whose husband had recently died of cancer. I tried to put it out of my mind but I couldn't. It would turn over and over in my head. I couldn't stop thinking that something was really wrong with me.'

Luckily this patient came for acupuncture treatment and in time the obsessive thoughts went away. When I saw her two years later she told me: 'I've stayed a lot stronger and have put on weight. I've also coped with two deaths. I very occasionally get a slight twinge in my breast but I don't worry about cancer any more.'

Another patient is typical of some people who worry and told me, 'I'm feeling much better and stronger than I was but I'm now worried about what will happen next – it's all going too well!'

Worry and its effect on your health

Emotional support can be very powerful in the face of worry. Research at Stanford University in the USA found that when groups of women who had advanced breast cancer unburdened their worries they lived twice as long as those who didn't. The only difference between these groups was that those who survived longest regularly attended meetings where they were with other women who had similar problems, and whom they knew were willing to listen to them.[15]

Joy

Joy is the final emotion I'll examine as a cause of disease. It is a rather surprising one as few patients come to me complaining of being too joyful!

Joy in the context of ill-health is not contentment and satisfaction, but is a more unsettled feeling that could sometimes be described as 'over-stimulation'. Too much joy affects the Heart.

Many people dream of winning the lottery but they might ask themselves, 'How would I really cope?' One sudden burst of euphoria has been known to cause a heart attack and certainly seems to lead to the opposite emotion of joylessness later on. Family break-ups, greed and sadness can often follow on the tail of this sudden joy. As it says in *Dao de Jing*, the original book of Daoism, 'To have enough is happiness. To have more than enough is harmful.'

As an acupuncturist, I find that I am more likely to see patients with the opposite problem – feeling joyless and miserable. Here a student tells me, 'I can get upset for a whole day when someone at college says something hurtful or if I feel I've said something I shouldn't. I feel quite miserable as I don't get on with people as well as I used to.'

After I treated this student he began to feel better. He was less vulnerable and hence could get on with other people more easily. He had found greater happiness in his life. The effect of treatment now will be important to his health in the future.

Are my emotions affecting my health?

1. Have you been under any prolonged or intense strain in your life that you still haven't recovered from?
2. Do you find it difficult to express your negative emotions?
3. Do you have a tendency to strong emotional feelings which you can't easily shrug off?
4. Is your current lifestyle causing you to feel stressed?

If the answer to at least two of these questions is Yes, then your emotions may be affecting your health.

More about internal causes of disease

ILLNESSES THAT CAN MANIFEST FROM AN INTERNAL CAUSE OF DISEASE

Many of the patients I see today have, at least to some degree, an emotional cause at the root of their illness. Almost any illness can result from an internal cause of disease. Although an emotional cause is frequently rooted in people's earliest childhood, the physical illness often doesn't manifest until much later on.

Certain conditions such as irritable bowel syndrome, stomach ulcers, heart conditions, insomnia and headaches are known to be exacerbated by people's emotional state but most other diseases can also have an internal cause. The imbalances which arise from your emotions can affect your body, mind and spirit depending on your current circumstances, constitution and lifestyle.

RESOLVING EMOTIONAL CAUSES

Acupuncture can strengthen the organs that have become weakened by internal causes. As treatment balances the Qi, patients often feel healthier and more able to deal with their feelings. Patients can feel increased well-being quite quickly and tell their acupuncturist that they feel better in themselves. This is a sign that the traumas of the past are starting to heal. Because emotional problems are sometimes very deep-seated changes tend to be more incremental and overall take longer to treat than external ones that are caused by pathogens.

The miscellaneous or lifestyle causes of disease

An unhealthy lifestyle can also affect our health. In the literal translation from Chinese these 'lifestyle' causes are called 'not internal and not external' causes of disease. They cover areas such as overwork and fatigue, exercise, diet and sex.

The importance of a healthy lifestyle

An in-depth study has been conducted into the lifestyle of many people in America over the last 30 years. It was carried out at the University of California School of Public Health and identified seven deadly health 'sins' that are likely to lead to an early and painful death.[16] They are:

- Obesity
- Physical inactivity
- Smoking
- Too much alcohol
- Sleeping too little or too much
- Eating irregularly
- Skipping breakfast.

In the study 7,000 adults were followed from the 1960s to the present day. It was found that these poor habits in combination could double the chance of dying prematurely or developing chronic illnesses.

Although smoking and alcohol were by far the deadliest of the 'sins', it was discovered that even slim, teetotal non-smokers whose only sins were to skip breakfast, eat between meals and sleep irregular hours were far more likely to suffer health problems or to die prematurely than those who led a healthier lifestyle. 'It seems that regularity of lifestyle must be health maintaining,' said Dr Breslow, who ran the study.

Lifestyle is important. Eating healthily and regularly, getting enough rest and exercise and protecting yourself from the elements will help you to remain healthy.

Diet

Everyone differs in their dietary needs. As a general rule eating three meals a day at regular times and without eating too late at night will maintain the efficient functioning of your digestive system.

Contrary to some current Western thought, Chinese medicine says that the Stomach and Spleen tend not to like too much uncooked or cold food, especially when the weather is cold. Warm cooked food is more easily transformed and digested than cold food. Iced food or drinks straight from the fridge take a great deal of energy to digest and are a definite 'no-no', especially in cold weather. For more on the temperature of food see page 196.

Keeping a good balance in the proportions of food you eat is also important. These proportions vary from individual to individual but on balance it is best to eat some grains, beans, fruit and vegetables, with smaller amounts of very nutritious foods such as meat, fish, eggs and dairy products. Flesh foods are important for your health but are classed as very 'rich' and as such should not be eaten in large quantities. It is also important to get enough oil in your diet. For example, organic cold pressed olive oil or flax oil can be added to vegetables and other food.

Ancient Chinese doctors – *Sun Si Miao* and his treatments

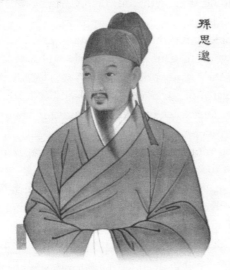

Sun Si Miao (pronounced 'Sun See Me-ow') was a doctor and a Buddhist who spent much of his life in seclusion. He lived during the Tang dynasty roughly between AD 582 and 682. He was asked to act as the personal physician to two different emperors of China and refused on each occasion, saying that he preferred to treat ordinary people. He learned to treat many common ailments concerned with nutrition and prescribed special diets for certain diseases. For example, he correctly recommended foods rich in iodine such as kelp, seaweed, and lamb and deer thyroid for a condition known as goitre, which is a swelling of the thyroid gland. He also cured an illness now known as beri beri, which is

95

due to a lack of vitamin B, by prescribing foods such as wheatgerm, liver and almonds.

Work and rest

As a rule of thumb, for every three hours of work we should have an hour's relaxation. This can include socialising with friends, spending time with your family, having a gentle walk, reading or talking.

Many people push themselves way beyond their natural capacity to work. In China, most people will have a rest after lunch before they start working again. A small study in the UK has shown that more accidents take place between 2 pm and 4 pm than at any other time in the day. Our brains are programmed for sleep not only at night but also after lunch. This makes driving more hazardous and can have repercussions on the quality of the work that people do.

Nowadays many people work through their lunch breaks and on into the afternoon – often on a diet of sandwiches and other cold foods. The saying that 'all work and no play makes Jack a dull boy (or Jill a dull girl)' is just as important now as it was in our grandmothers' day!

Exercise

Finding a balance between too much exercise and too little varies from individual to individual and taking notice of your body's needs is very important. Too much exertion can be just as bad for you as not exercising at all. People have been known to over-stimulate themselves to the point of collapse because they are obsessed by fitness – on some rare occasions this can be fatal.

The problems caused by too little activity are just as bad. Studies have found that children are taking one-third less exercise than they did in the 1930s. Research at Exeter University in Devon has found that nearly one-third of the ten-year-old girls and one in five of the boys studied were so inactive that they did not even manage a brisk ten-minute walk during the one week in which they were monitored. Because they were taking so little exercise, children were eating nearly one-third less in calories than they did 60 years ago yet they were more overweight![17]

In these days of increased car use, more television and computer games children easily miss out on exercise. Activity needs to be encouraged more strenuously to prevent young people establishing dangerous habits for their future.

Sex

Chinese medicine recognised that too much or too little sex can be a cause of disease and warned that this is especially important for men rather than women. Men can wear out their Kidney Essence if they ejaculate too often. This can result in possible back problems, tiredness and premature ageing. The issue of what exactly is too much sex has been much debated in many texts throughout Chinese history. There is a natural balance between too much and too little sex. Too little sex can lead to frustration and resentment, also possibly causing illness.

When people are ill, they need to cut down on their sexual activity to help them regain their health. Some people naturally have less desire to have sex when they are ill or overworking and this is normal. Many Chinese texts give guidelines about sexual activity when people are unwell, and discuss what constitutes a normal level of sexual activity at different stages in our lives. All the ancient Chinese doctors had different opinions, however! In general it is normal for younger people to enjoy a more active sex life and for this to decline steadily as a person gets older. As a rule of thumb, a maximum frequency of ejaculation for a man in good health at the age of 20 would be twice a day, at 30 once a day, at 40 every three days, at 50 every five days, at 60 every ten days and at 70 every thirty days. This should be halved if the person is unwell or tired. Sexual activity also changes with the seasons. It is normal to enjoy more sex during the summer when it is hotter and have less sexual activity in the colder months.

Is my lifestyle healthy?

- Do you eat three meals a day including breakfast?

- Do you eat at regular times and not too late in the evening?

- Do you chew your food?

- Do you normally eat generous amounts of fresh, cooked vegetables and fruit on a daily basis?

- Do you follow a two-thirds work to one-third rest ratio?

- Do you get enough rest time and breaks at work?

- Do you sleep for at least eight hours and go to bed at a regular time?

- Do you exercise regularly and in a balanced way (ie not over- or under-exercise)?

If you answered yes to most of these questions then your lifestyle is generally healthy.

The internal, external and miscellaneous causes of disease can all have an impact on your health. Caring for yourself by balancing your diet, exercise, work and rest can have a huge impact on your overall health. Simple lifestyle changes can enable you to maintain your health. The healthier you are the less you are affected by pathogens of Wind, Cold, Damp, Heat and Dryness – and protecting yourself from these pathogens can also be important. The internal (emotional) causes of disease often lie at the root of a person's health problems, however, as they frequently arise at an early stage in a person's life.[18]

Summary

- Chinese medicine describes three main factors that cause disease. These are:
  - External causes which are due to climate
  - Internal causes which are due to emotions
  - Miscellaneous or 'lifestyle' causes.
- The greater understanding people have of the causes of disease, the more they can do to protect themselves.
- The external causes of disease are Cold, Damp, Wind, Heat and Dryness. These causes of disease strongly correlate with 'old wives' tales' that many people were taught as children.
- If an illness has given rise to symptoms of Cold, Damp, Wind, Heat, or Dryness, treatments can be planned specifically to clear them from the body.
- The internal causes of disease are anger, grief, fear and shock, worry, over-thinking and joy. Although Chinese medicine named these seven emotions they include all other emotions.
- The roots of the internal causes of disease are often established at an early age and arise when a child experiences prolonged, intense, unexpressed or unresolved emotional states.
- Acupuncture can strengthen the Organs that have become weakened by the internal causes of disease and enable people's emotional problems to be resolved.

- The miscellaneous causes of disease are also called 'lifestyle' causes. They cover areas such as overwork and fatigue, exercise, diet and sex.
- Balancing these in your lifestyle can have a major impact on keeping you healthy.

6

The Theory of Chinese Medicine: Our Internal Map

The theoretical framework of Chinese medicine

When I first studied acupuncture I became familiar with many ancient Chinese doctors who are famous for the texts they wrote. In China, doctors traditionally refer back to and quote the writings of their predecessors, enabling them to build on and enrich the existing tradition and ensure it continues. The fact that these texts have been preserved for thousands of years is what has enabled Chinese medicine to survive to this day.

The most well-known acupuncture text is called *Huang Ti Nei Jing* (pronounced 'Hwang Chee Nay Jing') or The Yellow Emperor's Classic of Internal Medicine. In this text the Yellow Emperor has an interesting dialogue with his physician Qi Bo (pronounced 'Chee Bo'). The conversation covers all the basic theories of Chinese medicine. This text was written around 200 BC. Much of the acupuncture theory taught today is rooted in this book and it is still referred to extensively.

In this chapter I will discuss this underlying theory and how it is still as relevant to our health today as it was all of those years ago.

Ancient Chinese doctors – the Yellow Emperor and the *Huang Ti Nei Jing*

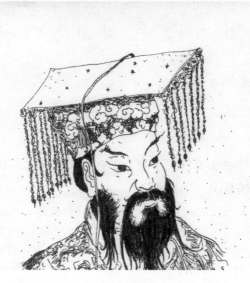

The Yellow Emperor is thought to have reigned between 2767 and 2696 BC. Although the *Huang Ti Nei Jing* text is attributed to him, subsequent research has shown that this book was actually written nearer to 200 BC. The information has been handed down and synthesised over centuries. To get an idea of the importance of this work to Chinese medicine you could compare it to the complete works of Shakespeare in English literature, or of Plato in philosophy. It is much quoted by all scholars and doctors of Chinese medicine to back up their own theories.

The Yellow Emperor's Classic of Internal Medicine is made up of two books, the *Su Wen* or 'Simple Questions' and the *Ling Shu* or 'Miraculous Pivot'. Chinese scholars have now discovered that these books were written not by one, but by many different writers who all wished to have their work attributed to this renowned doctor so as to give weight to their discoveries via the venerated *Huang Ti*.

How doctors attributed their works in China at that time is a curious reversal of the way things are now carried out in the Western world. Here, desire for success means that people like to have whatever they have created clearly attributed to themselves. Chinese doctors at that time were obviously more dedicated to the truth than to becoming famous!

The acupuncturist's toolbox

In order to make an accurate diagnosis of your health, practitioners have many tools in their 'toolbox'. One of the principal tools is the understanding of Yin and Yang and how their balance affects your health. Knowledge of the Vital Substances, the Five Elements and the 12 Organs or 'Officials' is also an essential part of this underlying theory. Finally, the pathogens such as Wind, Cold, Damp, Heat and Dryness that were described in the previous chapter also contribute to the practitioner's understanding of your condition. When used together all of these tools enable your practitioner to make a diagnosis by creating a complete picture of the state of your health.

Yin and Yang

The meaning of Yin and Yang

Chinese medicine describes every interaction in the universe in terms of Yin and Yang. The *Huang Ti Nei Jing*, the text discussed above, describes how important they are:

> *To live in harmony with Yin and Yang means life.*
> *To live against Yin and Yang means death.*
> *To live in harmony with Yin and Yang will bring peace.*
> *To live against Yin and Yang will bring chaos.*[1]

Yin and Yang represent the two fundamental forces of the universe. The Chinese character for Yang means 'the sunny side of

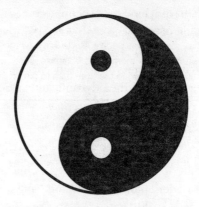

the hill' while the character for Yin depicts 'the shady side of the hill'. Chinese characters are an ideographic 'picture' that convey a vivid image of the meaning of the words they describe.

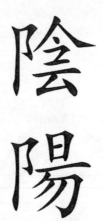

The four characteristics of Yin and Yang

Thirty years ago the words Yin and Yang were hardly understood in the West at all. Now they are so well known that they are almost a part of our everyday language. Most people, however, think of Yin and Yang as two opposing forces, just like sunshine and shade or light and dark. Although that is partially true there is far more to the two forces.

Chinese medicine describes four main characteristics of Yin and Yang in order to explain their dynamic interaction. They are:

> *Yin and Yang are in opposition.*
> *Yin and Yang are interdependent.*
> *Yin and Yang consume each other.*
> *Yin and Yang transform into each other.*

The sunny and shady sides of the hill

The image of the sunny and shady sides of the hill depicts the above four aspects very clearly.

Where there is sunshine there must be shade; each is conditional on the other's presence and they cannot be separated. As well as being in opposition, Yin and Yang are also said to be interdependent. As the days and seasons change, the quantities

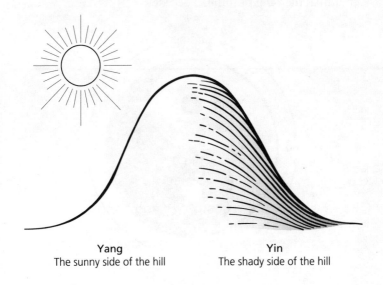

Yang
The sunny side of the hill

Yin
The shady side of the hill

of sunshine and shade are constantly changing in their relationship. In the morning the sun rises and as the day continues the amount of brightness increases while the shade lessens. As the evening descends the shade begins to increase again until the sun finally sets. The image depicts how Yin and Yang consume each other. Night-time is more Yin and daytime more Yang. The balance of Yin and Yang is never static; each one is constantly transforming into the other.

The relativity of Yin and Yang

Everything in the universe can be described in terms of Yin and Yang, so it is important to understand that the two principles are relative. A day is only one small part of the whole year, which also has Yin and Yang qualities. For instance, during the year the summer (which is brighter and hotter) is more Yang in quality and the winter (which is colder and darker) is more Yin. When spring arises, the Yin of winter declines, reappearing in autumn as the Yang of summer recedes.

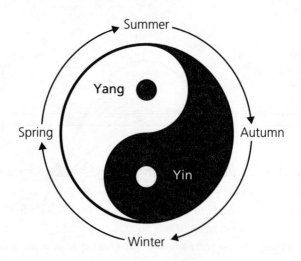

The balance of Yin and Yang is also important in the practice of acupuncture.

Some Yin and Yang characteristics

Each of us has our own particular balance of Yin and Yang. Yang is associated with **fire**; in other words it is dry, bright, hot, active and moving upwards and outwards. Yin can be characterised as associated with **water** as in a deep lake; in other words it is wet, dark and deep, cold and still.

Some Yin and Yang properties

Yin	Yang
Water	Fire
Cold	Heat
Wet	Dry
Interior	Exterior
Passive	Active
Slow	Rapid
Descending	Rising
Below	Above
Feminine	Masculine
Soft	Hard
Front	Back
Contraction	Expansion

How the concept of Yin and Yang is useful to an acupuncturist

When you become ill the balance of your Yin and Yang is affected. If you become hotter in temperature, over-active, feel drier in your body and become hotter tempered, your illness is more Yang in nature. Your fire is starting to rage and is not held in check by your Yin. This may result in many different symptoms ranging from hot flushes to fevers, dark scanty urine, constipation and restlessness.

On the other hand you may have too much Yin Qi, which is not being kept in check by your Yang Qi. In this case, you may retain more body fluid, slow down and become very tired. You might also experience symptoms such as chills, profuse pale urine, diarrhoea, lethargy or depression.

The Yin and Yang cycle in your life

At the beginning of our lives we are normally very Yang. We move from being energetic children to active adults. Later in life we naturally become more Yin and may wish to slow down. It is very common in the West for people to ignore any signs of ageing. We are encouraged to fight nature rather than work with it. As a result, many people work too hard when they should be resting. They can thus become deficient in Yin energy later in life.

This is especially true of women who at the time of the menopause become hotter, dryer and sometimes more restless – all signs of the Yin energy becoming depleted. It is interesting to note that hot flushes are less common in China, where women are more aware of their Yin nature in the latter part of their life, than in the West.

When an acupuncturist examines a patient, she or he assesses the relative balance between the patient's Yin and Yang. Knowing this, and with regard to the functioning of the 'vital substances' the practitioner can then prescribe treatment to re-establish better equilibrium, thus restoring health.

How balanced is my Yin and Yang?

1. Do you prefer a temperature that is: (a) hot; (b) cold; (c) a balance of the two?

2. When you feel tired do you: (a) keep on working when you know you should stop; (b) find you stop at the drop of a hat and can't start again; (c) feel refreshed after a rest?

3. If you get frustrated do you: (a) become easily irritated or angry; (b) withdraw and become depressed; (c) stay balanced and handle the situation well?

4. Do you perspire: (a) a lot and/or more at night; (b) not very much and/or more during the day; (c) a balanced amount with normal activity?

5. Does your urine tend to be: (a) scanty and dark; (b) pale and profuse; (c) more or less normal?

6. In social situations do you: (a) tend to be talkative; (b) prefer to stay quiet; (c) neither, I keep a happy medium?

7. In general are you: (a) a lark; (b) a night owl; (c) neither?

More (a) answers indicate that you are more Yang, more (b) answers indicate that you are more Yin. More (c) answers mean you are well balanced. A mixture of answers means you have both Yin and Yang signs.

The vital substances

What are the vital substances?

Western medicine describes the cell as the essential structural unit of the human body. Physiology is the science of the body's 'normal' functioning. The vital substances are the equivalent in Chinese medicine. These substances are created in the Yin Organs (see Chapter 7) and are the main constituents of a person. Their functioning could be described as 'Chinese physiology'.

The vital substances are:

- Qi
- Essence
- Blood
- Body Fluids
- Shen or Spirit.

Qi

WHAT IS QI?

Qi is the energy that underlies everything in the universe. If it is condensed it becomes matter or if refined it becomes spirit. The Chinese character for Qi shows the 'vapour' or 'gas' given off during the cooking of rice.

Qi is variously called *ki* in Japan, *prana* in India and *rlun* in Tibet. It has also been translated in various other ways including 'influences', 'life force', 'breath' or 'vital energy'.

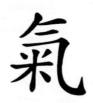

To a practitioner of Chinese medicine the theory of Qi is important. If you tried to see particles of Qi through a microscope you would not find it, but the restoration of its balance is vital to restore a patient's health. Everything that is living, moving and vibrating does so because this invisible substance moves through it. The reason that your blood circulates, your limbs move, your stomach digests food and your hair grows is because you have Qi activating everything in your body. Your Qi gives you vitality. Without it you would no longer be alive.

The Qi inside your body is created from the combination of the food you eat and digest via your Stomach and Spleen and the air you breathe into your Lungs. In fact Chinese medicine considers Qi to be so important that a Chinese text called the *Nan Jing* states: 'Qi is the root of all human beings.'

THE FUNCTIONS OF QI

Qi has five main functions. It moves, transforms, protects, warms and holds or contains.

Qi and movement. Qi creates all involuntary and voluntary movement such as the beating of your heart, the continuation of breathing while you sleep and the ability to move your body from place to place or your thoughts from subject to subject.

Qi and transformation. Qi enables your food to be assimilated, air to oxygenate your blood and information to be taken in and digested. All processing in the body and mind comes about as a result of the Qi's transformative function.

Qi and protection. Your defensive Qi allows you to have a strong immune system, leading to the ability to resist diseases. If people easily succumb to infections this may be because their protective Qi is weak.

Qi and warming. Qi keeps your blood at a stable temperature. Humans are warm-blooded and warmth is essential to the maintenance of good health.

Qi and containment. Qi allows all of your Organs, tissues and blood vessels to remain in their correct position in the body, ensuring their continued ability to function healthily.

DISHARMONIES OF QI

If Qi goes out of balance it becomes either deficient or stagnant.

Deficient Qi. If your Qi becomes deficient this will result in an inability to remain vital and energetic throughout the day. If plants are not nourished they wilt. Without enough Qi you can also wilt and feel increasingly feeble. As a result you can easily become depleted and lethargic and will not have enough energy to get through the day. Other symptoms include breathlessness, especially on exertion, a weak voice, poor appetite and spontaneous sweating.

Deficient Qi can also cause 'sinking Qi'. This can lead to prolapsed Organs because the Qi no longer holds them in their correct position.

Most people who are ill have some underlying Qi deficiency although it may not be the main reason for their problem. For example, Samantha, who had post-viral syndrome, lay on the sofa for five years when she was very ill – Qi deficiency was one of many aspects of her diagnosis. The same is true of Francesca, who reported that her energy levels were very low before she had acupuncture.

Stagnant Qi. If the normal flow of Qi becomes blocked this is called 'stagnant Qi'. Stagnant Qi often occurs in a limb if you injure yourself. In this case the instinctive need to rub the area will enable your Qi to move once more. Qi also stagnates when you hold back your emotions, especially anger. In this case you could have a variety of different symptoms that include depression or mood swings, pre-menstrual tension, digestive problems, and a lump or 'plumstone' throat. These symptoms can all be caused when people do not express themselves.

If food, fluid or breath becomes blocked or travels in the wrong direction this is called 'rebellious Qi' and can cause symptoms such as vomiting, belching or a cough.

How balanced is my Qi?

1. Do you often feel tired or tire towards the end of the day even without overdoing it?
2. Do you find it a strain to assert yourself?
3. If you're feeling tired do you find it hard to digest your food or do you easily get loose bowels?
4. Do you sometimes feel weak in your legs and prefer to sit down?
5. Do you easily feel breathless, especially if you exert yourself, eg run for a short distance?

If the answer to at least two of the questions above is Yes then you may have a tendency towards Qi deficiency.

1. Do you sometimes feel really tired, then go for a run or exercise and feel instantly better?
2. Do others describe you as moody, or if you are a woman do you often get pre-menstrual tension?
3. Do you get depressed, then feel better if you go out and socialise?
4. Do you have symptoms that seem to move around or come and go?
5. Do you sometimes have a feeling of distension in your chest, ribcage or abdomen?

If the answer to at least two of the questions above is Yes then you may have a tendency towards Qi stagnation.

Essence

WHAT IS ESSENCE?

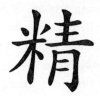

You inherit your Essence (or Constitutional Essence as it is sometimes called) from your parents. The strength of it determines the robustness of your constitution. Chinese medicine teaches that it is stored in the Kidneys and allows you to develop from childhood to adulthood and then into old age. Children reach puberty, then mature until they can conceive and have children. At the end of their fertile lives women go through the menopause and stop menstruating. Chinese medicine teaches that the ability to move through these different stages and cycles of our lives is due to this Essence.

ESSENCE AND YOUR HEALTH

The Essence that you inherit at birth is the quantity that you have for the rest of your life. Some people are frail from birth or have slightly slower mental or physical development than is normal. Although they may be slightly deficient in Essence, if they conserve their energy carefully they can live long and happy lives. Some illnesses termed 'congenital' may also be due to deficient Essence.

This Constitutional Essence gives us a natural 'moistness'. We see this in new born infants and young children. As we age, we start to dry up. Greying hair, falling teeth, wrinkling skin, stiff joints and failing memories are all signs that the Essence is becoming depleted. Ageing is a natural process, but the more care you put into looking after your overall health the better you conserve your Essence later in life.

A STRONG CONSTITUTION

Most people have an average amount of Essence. There is no situation in which people have too much Essence – those people with exceptionally strong constitutions are just called lucky!

Chinese medicine teaches some other ways to assess the overall strength of your constitution:

- your overall stamina
- the length of your earlobes
- the strength of your jaw line.

A useful way of assessing the strength of our constitution is to consider our overall robustness. If we have a lot of stamina, a naturally strong physique and can easily work hard and recover our energy quickly, this may indicate that we have strong Constitutional Essence.

Ancient Chinese texts also talk about the size of the ears and the length of the earlobes as a guide to the strength of the Essence. The ears should be well placed – that is, not too high on the head. They should be a good size in relation to the person's build. The earlobes should also be long.[2]

If we look at Oriental pictures of the Buddha, he is often depicted as having huge earlobes – signifying the extraordinary strength of his essence. While long and full lobes are said to indicate a strong constitution, small thin earlobes are said to indicate a less strong one.

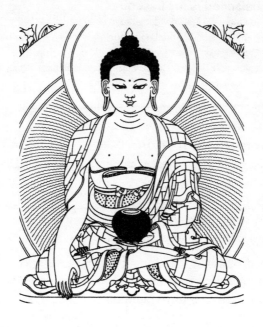

A strong jaw line will indicate the strength of the constitution. It is interesting to note that if people have interbred, the offspring will, over generations, develop smaller and weaker chins and jaw lines. This indicates their decreased strength and weakened constitutions.

TREATMENT FOR ESSENCE DEFICIENCY

Our constitutional strength is difficult to change so extreme problems caused by Essence deficiencies can be hard to treat. Acupuncture treatment on the Kidneys (which store the Essence) can, however, strengthen a person with slightly deficient Essence and generally prevent problems from developing.[3]

How balanced is my Essence?

1. Do you regularly feel very depleted in energy?
2. Do you have signs of premature ageing, such as greying hair, baldness, drying skin or wrinkles?
3. Have you had difficulty conceiving, continuous backaches, an early menopause if you are a woman or impotence or a low sperm count if you are a man?
4. Are you constantly getting infections and do you invariably catch other people's colds and flu?
5. Have you got small ears and short earlobes, or a weak jaw line?

If the answer to three or more of these questions is Yes then you may have slightly deficient Essence.

Blood

Besides diagnosing the functioning of a person's Qi and Essence the practitioner also examines the state of the Blood. This flows with the Qi in the body. Qi and Blood are mutually dependent. Chinese medicine teaches that the Qi moves the Blood so that it stays in the Blood vessels and circulates throughout the body. In turn the Blood nourishes the Organs that produce the Qi.

WHAT DOES THE TERM 'BLOOD' MEAN?

To many of you, the question 'What is Blood?' will seem rather a silly one. It's the red fluid that flows through our arteries and veins, of course! In the practice of Chinese medicine, however, the Blood is described by what it *does* rather than by what it *is*.

Although Blood is, of course, the fluid that flows through your arteries and veins, in Chinese medicine it also has other functions.

THE FUNCTIONS OF BLOOD

The Blood has three main functions:

- to moisten
- to nourish
- to house the Shen or mind–spirit.

Nourishing and moistening. The Blood nourishes all parts of our body. This includes the muscles, tendons and ligaments, as well as the eyes, skin, hair and complexion.

Housing the Shen or mind–spirit. Blood is a much 'heavier' substance than Qi. If you have sufficient Blood the most refined part of you – your mind–spirit – can rest peacefully in the Heart. This allows people to feel calm and settled, have a good memory and a strong sense of self-worth.

DISHARMONIES OF BLOOD

When the Blood becomes imbalanced it can become deficient, stagnant or too hot.

Blood deficiency. In my acupuncture practice I very commonly see patients with signs and symptoms of Blood deficiency. When Westerners hear the term 'Blood deficiency' they often associate it with anaemia – a symptom that occurs when your red blood cell count becomes low. Blood deficiency doesn't mean that you are anaemic, however. The signs and symptoms may include anaemia but are far wider ranging.

Symptoms of Blood deficiency include frequent pins and needles or cramps due to malnourishment of the muscles and tendons, or dry skin and eyes, brittle nails and aching joints due to insufficient moistening of the extremities. Constant anxiety, poor memory, a lack of concentration and poor sleep can also occur due to the Blood not 'housing' the Shen. A person who is Blood deficient often has a dull, pale complexion and a woman may have scanty periods.

Blood deficiency may be caused by heavy bleeding and is especially common in women who have heavy periods or lose a lot of blood while giving birth. It can also be caused by a diet lacking in protein or by excessive anxiety. Jenny, who in Chapter 2 told us about her anxiety resulting from the stress of her exams, had Blood deficiency. Besides anxiety some of her other symptoms were poor sleep, lack of concentration and a pale, dull complexion.

Blood stagnation. Symptoms of Blood stagnation arise when the Blood is not flowing smoothly. This can cause sharp or stabbing pain (such as some period pains) or masses such as fibroids and lumps.

Heat in the Blood. If the Blood becomes overheated it can lead to symptoms of bleeding such as uterine haemorrhage or nosebleeds.

TREATING THE BLOOD

When people have problems with their Blood, acupuncture can help to create a better state of health. Lifestyle changes, such as eating more protein in the diet, can also be useful. For more on this see Chapter 9.

How balanced is my Blood?

1. Do your nails break easily?
2. Do you frequently get cramps or pins and needles in your limbs?
3. Do you startle or get anxious easily or have a poor memory?
4. If you are a woman, do you have scanty periods that last no more than three days?
5. Do you often find it hard to get off to sleep, or do you sleep lightly?
6. Do you feel slightly light-headed when moving from sitting to standing?

If the answer to three or more of these questions is Yes then you may be slightly Blood deficient.

The Body Fluids

WHAT ARE BODY FLUIDS?

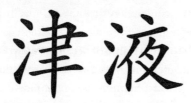

'Jin Ye' is the term used in Chinese medicine to describe all the fluids in the body.

The Jin Body Fluids are light and watery and are at the exterior of our body. They nourish the skin and muscles and come out as sweat, saliva and mucus. The Ye Body Fluids are heavier and are contained more within our bodies. They moisturise the joints, the brain, the spine and the bone marrow. When your Body Fluids are balanced they flow smoothly through the body and allow all areas of your body to be well lubricated.

DISHARMONIES OF BODY FLUIDS

If the Body Fluids are deficient a person becomes dehydrated. If they get stuck and are not moving smoothly around the body, they may be retained and cause either 'Damp', oedema or 'Phlegm' in the body.

Heavy thighs or the formation of a paunch can be due to stuck Body Fluids, known by the Chinese as 'Damp'.[4] Other symptoms of Damp include a heavy head, heavy limbs, sluggishness and poor concentration. Oedema in the body is also due to retained Body Fluids and leads to swollen limbs and bloating.

Phlegm can also be formed when Body Fluids are stuck. This can manifest as phlegm in the nose or chest. Chinese medicine describes many other symptoms that are caused by Phlegm. These include lumps under the skin, bone or joint deformities, and stones in the gall bladder or kidneys.

TREATMENT FOR BODY FLUID DISHARMONIES

The Spleen transforms and transports everything in the body (see Chapter 7) and treatment to the Spleen can be a very important way of moving Body Fluids. If the Body Fluids are stuck this can obstruct the free movement of the Qi and Blood in the body.

The Body Fluids are the most 'substantial' of all of the Substances in the body. This is in contrast to the Shen, roughly translated as 'Mind–Spirit', which is the most 'insubstantial'.

How balanced are my Body Fluids?

1. Do you sometimes feel heavy in your limbs or head?
2. Do you get large amounts of catarrh or cough up phlegm in the mornings?
3. Do you easily retain Body Fluids and get swelling in your feet, legs or ankles?
4. Do you easily bloat up in your abdomen or stomach?
5. Do you ever feel extremely sluggish and have difficulty concentrating?

If the answer to three or more of these questions is Yes then you may be prone to retaining Body Fluids.

The Shen or Spirit

WHAT IS SHEN?

Shen could be said to be a very rarefied form of Qi, but it could also be called your mind-spirit. It is housed in the Heart by the Blood. The Shen is said to be so refined and light that it needs the Blood, which is a heavier substance, to keep it settled in place.

BALANCED SHEN

If your Shen is settled you will be calm and centred and unruffled by problems or setbacks. You will also sleep well, think clearly, and have a good memory and a strong sense of purpose in your life. It will also show itself by a bright shine in your eyes.

DISHARMONIES OF SHEN

Shen can be imbalanced in three main ways. It can be:

- Disturbed
- Deficient
- Obstructed.

Disturbed Shen. Many people have some disturbance in their Shen. This can be short term if you have a physical or emotional shock. Or it can be more long term if your Blood is deficient or your Heart is weakened. Difficulties that arose during childhood can affect people deeply and cause problems that affect their mind–spirit later in life.

If your Shen is disturbed you can become anxious, jumpy, lacking in concentration and possibly have difficulty sleeping. You may also startle easily and have palpitations at night. These signs and symptoms occur because your Shen is unable to rest if your Heart Blood is deficient.

Deficient Shen. The Shen may be deficient, causing a person to feel dull, apathetic, depressed and lacking in spirit.

Obstructed Shen. Obstruction of the Shen is less common and can cause more severe problems. In the two situations above, the Shen's ability to settle tends to come and go. If it is obstructed it is blocked and unable to settle in its resting place. This can cause a person to have a clouded mind and symptoms of mania, such as being unable to sleep, constantly hyperactive, confused and out of control of their actions.[5]

TREATING THE SHEN

Acupuncture is often used to treat problems affecting the Shen. Sometimes changes can be almost instantaneous. When problems go back to early childhood, longer-term treatment may be required.

How balanced is my Shen?

1. Do you have problems getting off to sleep or do you wake during the night?
2. Do you have a poor short-term memory and easily forget things?
3. Do you tend to startle easily or feel jumpy for no reason?
4. Do you easily get anxious and/or go over and over things in your mind?
5. Do you have a low sense of self-esteem or lack purpose in your life?

If the answer to three or more of these questions is Yes then you may have some Shen disturbance.

The Three Treasures

The Qi, the Essence and the Shen are called 'the Three Treasures'. Together they are the basis of all energetic transformations in the body. In Chinese medicine the term 'Jingshen' (Jing is the Chinese word for Essence) is often used as a shorthand term for vitality or vigour, indicating the understanding that a good constitution and a strong spirit are the basis of a healthy life.

Alongside Yin and Yang and the vital substances, a knowledge of the Five Elements and their 12 Organs are an important part of diagnosis. These will be discussed in the next chapter.

Summary

- In order to make an accurate diagnosis, practitioners have many tools in their toolbox. These include knowledge of Yin and Yang and the vital substances, the Organs and the Five Elements.

- Yin and Yang represent the two fundamental forces of the universe. An acupuncturist strives to bring balance to a patient's Yin or Yang Qi when it is out of balance.

- The vital substances are the main constituents of a person. They interact together in order that a person can have energy and vitality. The substances are Qi, Essence, Blood, Body Fluids and Shen (or Spirit).

- When the substances are depleted or blocked, acupuncture can be used to restore their balance.

- The Qi, Essence and Shen together form 'the Three Treasures'. Chinese medicine considers that their healthy functioning forms the basis for a strong constitution, a strong mind and spirit and therefore a healthy life.

7

The 12 Organs and Officials: In the Emperor's Court

An introduction to the Organs and Officials

Chinese medicine emphasises an Organ's wider energetic functions and describes them more poetically than Western medicine. For example, Western medicine describes the heart as a pump for the blood. In comparison, Chinese medicine describes how the Heart has control over your whole circulatory system – right down to the smallest capillary. It goes on further to compare the Heart to an Emperor. In ancient times the Emperor of China was the supreme controller of the whole country. Similarly, the Heart is the 'supreme controller' of a person. This is because it houses your Shen or mind-spirit, thus influencing your ability to be calm, clear-thinking and joyful.

Chinese medicine describes how the Lungs preside over the whole of the respiratory system, including the nose and the trachea and also your ability to express grief. Not only do the

Lungs affect your ability to breathe in air, they are also the 'Receivers of Qi from the Heavens' and enable you to revitalise your Qi.

In a similar way physical, mental and emotional qualities are also ascribed to the other Organs. Consequently, Chinese medical treatment often affects you in a broader way than you might expect and can influence your health psychologically as well as physically.

The Organs and their functions

The 12 Organs are divided into six Yin Organs and six Yang Organs. Each Yin Organ is paired with a Yang Organ and each Organ is connected to a channel or pathway of Qi, as described in Chapter 4.

The Yin and Yang Organs

Yin Organ	Liver	Heart	Pericardium	Spleen	Lung	Kidneys
Yang Organ	Gall Bladder	Small Intestine	Triple Burner	Stomach	Large Intestine	Bladder

The Yin Organs are called solid Organs (you may wonder about the Lungs – they are much more solid than you think!) and have functions to do with the manufacture, storage and regulation of the vital substances that were described in the previous chapter. The Yang Organs are called hollow Organs (notice that they are all tubes or bags) and their functions have more to do with receiving, separating and distributing substances.

The Yin Organs lie deeper inside the body and have more functions than the Yang Organs. Both are important to the acupuncturist when carrying out treatment. Each Yin Organ is linked with a number of different areas of functioning and is associated with:

- One of the vital substances (Qi, Essence, Blood, Body Fluids and Shen, described in Chapter 6)
- A mind/spirit aspect
- A tissue
- A sense organ
- A body part.

The Organs and the Elements

Each pair of Organs is also associated with an Element (there are four Organs for the Fire Element). The Elements and their associated Yin and Yang Organs are:

ELEMENT	ORGANS
Wood	Liver and Gall Bladder
Fire	Heart and Small Intestine
	Pericardium and Triple Burner
Earth	Spleen and Stomach
Metal	Lung and Large Intestine
Water	Kidneys and Bladder

The Water Element, for example, relates to the Kidneys and the Bladder, both of which are associated with the assimilation of water in our bodies. The Earth Element is connected with the Spleen and Stomach. Food grows on the earth, so there is an obvious relationship between those Organs and that Element.

The Organs described as 'Officials'

The Organs are described in a very special way in Chapter 8 of the *Su Wen*. The *Su Wen* is part of the ancient text called the *Huang Ti Nei Jing*, which I talked about in Chapter 6. In this text each of the 12 Organs is described metaphorically as an 'Official' in the Emperor's court. Each has its own special job in running the 'country' and plays a part working in a team with the other Officials. As well as the Emperor, which is the Heart, other Officials include the prime minister (the Lungs) and the general (the Liver), right down to the rubbish collector (the Large Intestine).

The Organs working as a 'team'

Nowadays it might be more relevant to compare the Organs/Officials to a team working together in an office. All members of the team have their specific duties. Team members include the company director, the managers, the administration team and the office cleaners and caretakers. When they all work in harmony the office runs smoothly.

If one of the team can't work for a period of time everyone else comes under strain. The other team members take on the extra responsibilities in order to keep things running smoothly and they start to feel overloaded. The smooth functioning of the team starts to break down and they may bicker or become upset. If the person who is sick is supported until she or he is well again the whole team will settle and be able to work in harmony once more. This is the same if you are unwell. If the sick Organ is supported and restored to health all of your other Organs can relax and become healthier. Your internal 'team' will then work together and in harmony. Each of the Organs is described below.

The Liver and Gall Bladder (Wood)

The Liver – the planner

'The Liver is the general who works out the plans.'

Su Wen, Chapter 8[1]

The Liver is often compared to a military strategist or general because when it is working well it excels in the ability to think up plans and put them into action. In this way, it is a very creative Organ that enables you to assert yourself and move forward in order to fulfil your life's purpose.

PHYSICAL SIGNS AND SYMPTOMS

The Liver has many responsibilities to do with your Qi and Blood. First, it has the job of 'smoothing' the flow of your Qi. This is less to do with the overall quantity of your Qi and more to do with ensuring that it moves freely and easily throughout your body, mind and spirit. If you are relaxed your Qi will flow smoothly. If you are angry or are suppressing your emotions you will probably hold your muscles tensely, causing the Qi to stagnate.

Stagnation of your Liver Qi can lead to a variety of symptoms such as headaches, abdominal pain, a stuffy feeling in the chest and flatulence. It can also lead to frustration, irritability, anger, mood swings and depression. If you are a woman, stagnant Liver Qi commonly causes pre-menstrual syndrome, with these emotional symptoms linked to painful breasts or a bloated abdomen. It can also cause irregular periods or period pain.

Acupuncture can have a profound effect on many of these symptoms as it spreads the Qi and allows it to flow easily and smoothly once more, easing out a tense mind as well as a tense body. (Qi stagnation is described in more detail in Chapter 6 on page 112.)

The Liver also 'stores the Blood'. Chinese medicine states that when you are active the Blood flows to your extremities. When you are at rest the Blood then returns to the Liver. If your Blood is deficient it may be unable to flow to your extremities rapidly enough (the 'extremities' include your head). You will then have 'postural dizziness' for a short time as your Blood catches up with your movement. Other symptoms of Blood deficiency can be scanty periods, dry skin and hair, pins and needles and a pale complexion. The nails are described as the 'residue' of the Liver. If your nails break easily this may also indicate Liver Blood deficiency. (For more on Blood deficiency see Chapter 6, page 118.)

The eyes are the sense organ of the Liver, so if you have eye or vision problems such as dry or sore eyes, tense eyes, floaters (black spots in front of the eyes) or red eyes, the Liver may lie at the root of the problem. The Liver also affects your tendons and ligaments. If your Liver is healthy, your tendons will be healthy and supple. If it is stagnant, they may be tight and stiff. A deficient Liver is unable to nourish the tendons and ligaments and can cause signs and symptoms such as spasms and cramps, numbness or difficulty bending and stretching.

MENTAL AND EMOTIONAL FUNCTIONS AND SIGNS AND SYMPTOMS

Chinese medicine teaches that the Liver gives you the ability to make plans and decisions and have a sense of purpose in your life.

If you have a Liver imbalance you may have difficulty making plans. You may either compensate by over-planning or make no plans at all. Plans range from larger decisions such as what career to pursue, who to have a relationship with and where to live, to day-to-day considerations such as what to wear today, what to eat and what time to go to bed.

The Liver function also ensures that you grow towards fulfilling your life plan or destiny. Your life plan is not always something you are conscious of. It is often only experienced when it is missing and you have the uncomfortable sense that you are not moving towards your ultimate purpose or you don't have an overall sense of direction in life. Acupuncture treatment can help you regain a better balance of health, enabling you to regain the overview of this life plan.

The Gall Bladder – the decision-maker

'The Gall Bladder is responsible for what is just and exact. Determination and decision stem from it.'

Su Wen, Chapter 8

Just as the Liver is called 'the planner', the Gall Bladder, its paired Organ, is called 'the decision-maker'. It is responsible for making all of your decisions and judgements. Not surprisingly these two Organs work so closely together that they are almost inseparable.

PHYSICAL SIGNS AND SYMPTOMS

The Gall Bladder has the function of storing and secreting bile to aid digestion. If your Gall Bladder is not functioning well, you may have symptoms such as digestive problems, gallstones, headaches, nausea and eye problems. Women may also become clumsy around the time of their period if this Organ is not functioning well. This is partly because it controls your tendons (along with your Liver) and partly because of its job as your decision-maker. If your decision-maker is imbalanced you may have difficulties making decisions and judgements, and find it tricky to judge distances. The combined strain on these functions can cause co-ordination problems.

The Gall Bladder channel travels from the feet up the sides of the body to the head. Symptoms such as hip, flank (the sides), neck and shoulder problems can all result from obstruction in this channel.

MENTAL AND EMOTIONAL SIGNS AND SYMPTOMS

If you sometimes have difficulty making decisions this may be due to an imbalance in your Gall Bladder. Chinese medicine teaches that a healthy Gall Bladder enables you to make clear decisions based on sound judgement. An imbalanced Gall Bladder leads to indecision, vacillating or procrastinating or, at the other extreme, making badly thought-out snap decisions that are later regretted.

The Chinese have an expression that someone who is brave has a 'big Gall Bladder' while someone who is timid and can't assert themselves has a 'small Gall Bladder'.

How balanced are my Liver and Gall Bladder?

1. Do you often feel tense, frustrated and irritable or have mood swings or depression?
2. Do you ever get headaches or migraines?
3. Do you have pre-menstrual syndrome with any of the above emotional symptoms, as well as painful breasts or a bloated abdomen?
4. Do you have irregular periods, scanty periods or period pain?
5. Do you have postural dizziness, pins and needles, dry skin and hair and/or a pale complexion?
6. Do you get eye problems such as dry, sore eyes, tense eyes, floaters (black spots in front of the eyes) or red eyes?
7. Do you ever have problems with your ligaments and tendons, such as numbness or difficulty bending and stretching, or have co-ordination problems?

8. Do you ever have difficulty making plans and decisions?

If the answer to at least three of the questions above is Yes then you may have an imbalance in the Organs of the Wood Element – the Liver and Gall Bladder.

The Heart and Small Intestine (Fire)

The Heart – the supreme controller

> 'The Heart holds the office of lord and sovereign.
> The radiance of the spirit stems from it.'
>
> *Su Wen*, Chapter 8

Although all of your Organs are mutually dependent, the Heart or 'supreme controller' holds a place of prime importance. This is because, as I described above, in Chinese medicine the Heart is compared to an Emperor (you might also think of the chair of a board of directors). In China the Emperor was seen as half man and half divine. He was the people's connection to Heaven. If the Emperor was strong and ran the country fairly, peace prevailed in the land. If, on the other hand, the Emperor was weak, then chaos reigned. It is the same in your body. If the Heart does not function well then you may feel out of control, anxious or panicky.

PHYSICAL SIGNS AND SYMPTOMS

If your acupuncturist diagnoses that your Heart needs treatment this doesn't mean that you have a physical heart problem. Although some of the functions of the Heart overlap with the Western physiological functions, an acupuncturist can also treat your Heart for many other reasons, as you'll see below.

As both Chinese and Western medicine agree, one of the main functions of the Heart is to pump the blood around your body. Your Heart also presides over your blood vessels. It distributes nutrition and energy to every cell in your body, enabling you to remain energetic and vital. Symptoms arising from poor circulation, such as tiredness and cold hands and feet, may be treated via your Heart.

An acupuncturist can gauge the functioning of your Heart by looking at your complexion. If your Heart is strong then your complexion looks rosy and healthy; if your complexion looks more pale and dull this may indicate that the functioning of your Heart is deficient. Please note, however, a pale face does not mean that you have a physical heart problem in the Western medical sense.

The Heart opens into the tongue – in fact the Chinese call the tongue 'the offshoot of the Heart'. If your Heart is healthy you will be able to choose your words accurately in order to convey meaning and relate to others. If your Heart is slightly disturbed, this can sometimes make it difficult for you to express yourself through words. If you have a Heart imbalance you may sometimes be unable to find the right word or a wrong word may come out in place of the word you want.[2] Excessive laughing or giggling and loud speech can also indicate a Heart imbalance. Many speech defects such as stuttering or slurred speech can be helped by treating the Heart, as can problems with the tongue, such as ulcers and inflammation.

MENTAL AND EMOTIONAL FUNCTIONS AND SIGNS AND SYMPTOMS

The Chinese character for the Heart is very interesting. Rather than depicting a physical Organ, as most of the Chinese characters for an Organ do, it just depicts an empty space. The reason for this is that the Heart doesn't need to be active, rather it just needs to 'be' with a sense of spaciousness. People with healthy Hearts have a shine in their eyes and a glow in their faces which arise from the radiance of the mind-spirit shining through them.

The Heart is involved in making your Blood. Blood is a heavy substance while *Shen* is more refined. If your Heart Blood is not sufficient then your Shen will 'float'. A floating spirit makes you feel disturbed and you may then have symptoms such as anxiety, restlessness, agitation and/or panics. You may also have unsettled sleep, a poor memory and palpitations. (For more on the Shen and the Blood see Chapter 6.)

Because the Heart has an important effect on the Spirit, many emotions arise from it – especially joy and sorrow. Everyday expressions indicate this. Most of us understand from our own experience that a feeling of being 'heartbroken' is a very real and palpable sensation for someone who has just left a loving relationship and that a person who 'wears their heart on their sleeve' shows all of their feelings. If a person is 'heartened' by something it makes them feel cheerful, while a 'heartless' person is cruel and unloving. As well as giving you a sense of calmness, a healthy Heart gives you the ability to interact and make good contact with others.

The Small Intestine – the separator of pure from impure

> 'The Small Intestine is responsible for receiving and making things thrive. Transformed substances stem from it.'
>
> *Su Wen*, Chapter 8

The Small Intestine has been called the 'sorter' or 'separator of pure from impure' because it not only sorts out your physical food and fluids, but also your thoughts and feelings.

PHYSICAL SIGNS AND SYMPTOMS

The Small Intestine is a long, bag-like Organ that lies in your lower abdomen. Its physical functions are similar in both Chinese and Western medicine, in that it receives your digested food and drink from the Stomach. Chinese medicine describes it as then separating this out into the pure and the impure. It absorbs the pure and sends the impure to the Large Intestine for eventual evacuation. If your Small Intestine Organ is imbalanced you may have physical problems such as abdominal pain, intestinal rumblings, diarrhoea or constipation.

The Small Intestine channel starts on the little finger and runs along the arm and up the neck, to finish in front of the ear. Musculo-skeletal pains in the arm, shoulder blade, neck and ear can result from this channel being blocked or deficient.

MENTAL AND EMOTIONAL FUNCTIONS AND SIGNS AND SYMPTOMS

The Small Intestine, or 'sorter', can easily be affected mentally and emotionally – especially in the frantic twenty-first century. And the strain is increasing. As we are given more and more options in life, we need greater discrimination in order to weave our way through the maze of alternatives. For instance, think of all the choices we need to make in our lives – about relationships, holidays, job opportunities, health care, leisure activities, food, entertainment, what to wear – the list is endless. Then think of the constant bombardment we have from books, newspapers, TV, advertisements and films. All of this can take its toll on our Small Intestine.

At one time life was not necessarily easy but it was at least predictable and moved at a slow pace. Now the 'sorter' never stops as we go about our busy day-to-day lives. If people have an efficient 'sorter' they can easily decide what to take in and what to filter out, absorbing only the 'nutritious' parts of their interactions and activities.

If you have an imbalance in your Small Intestine you might find that you can easily get clogged with mental as well as physical debris. This can cause you to feel fuzzy and confused and make you unable to discriminate. For example, in a relationship a person might feel stuck in ambivalence – unable to commit themselves but unable to leave. A student writing an essay might find it hard to decide which information to keep and which to throw out, resulting in an essay that rambles and is twice as long as necessary. Another person might go to a disturbing film and be unable to sort and throw out unwanted thoughts and pictures from their head.

The Heart and Small Intestine at first sight appear to be an unusual pairing of Organs. If you consider that the Heart only needs to 'be', it is not so unusual. A well-functioning 'sorter' will protect the Heart by ensuring it throws out all unnecessary input, leaving it to 'run the country' in peace.

The Pericardium and Triple Burner (Fire)
The Pericardium – the Heart Protector

> 'The Pericardium represents the civil servants.
> From them come joy and pleasure.'
> *Su Wen*, Chapter 8

The Pericardium is sometimes called the 'Heart Protector'. The Heart's job of being a link between humanity and the universe is so important that it requires a protector.

PHYSICAL SIGNS AND SYMPTOMS
Western medicine describes the pericardium as a sheath or membrane that surrounds the heart. Chinese medicine

describes it in a similar way and says that it surrounds and protects the Heart. In Chinese medicine the symptoms of the Heart and the Pericardium are so close that an acupuncturist may need to treat a person who has 'Heart' symptoms on the Pericardium channel instead. Physically, the Pericardium can be the first line of defence when heat pathogens affect the Heart from the outside.

MENTAL AND EMOTIONAL FUNCTIONS AND SIGNS AND SYMPTOMS

In its role as the Heart Protector, the Pericardium functions rather like a gatekeeper to the Heart. The Heart Protector opens the gates and lets in any warmth and good feelings or closes them to keep out any hurts, insults and negativity. It would be impossible for an Emperor to see all of his subjects (or for the company director to see all of her/his clients). The job of the Heart Protector is to 'meet and greet', leaving the Emperor to preside over his realm.

If your Heart Protector is functioning well you have the strength to deal with any difficulties that come your way, especially in relationships. If your Heart Protector is imbalanced you may feel more vulnerable and may be either too open or too closed.

If a person is too open they may become over-sensitive, especially in close and intimate relationships, and may be hurt by what others would more easily shrug off. Alternatively, a person who is too closed might shut off their Heart to others and become withdrawn. As a result, they may have difficulties forming relationships, preferring to keep them more superficial, or being unable to take the constant hurts they feel as a result of being too open. If a person with this imbalance has acupuncture it can have a major effect on their stability and resilience, enabling them to open up and close down more appropriately and effectively.

The Triple Burner – the official of balance and harmony

> 'The Triple Burner is responsible for opening up passages and irrigation. The regulation of fluids stems from it.'
>
> *Su Wen*, Chapter 8

The Triple Burner is different from the other 11 Organs. That's because it's not really an organ at all! Rather, it is a division of the torso into three separate 'spaces' or 'burners'. It has the function of regulating the passage of Qi and Fluids through the Organs – in other words it keeps everything in balance and harmony.

PHYSICAL SIGNS AND SYMPTOMS

The three burners of the body lie on your torso. The upper burner lies at the level of the chest and affects your Heart, Pericardium and Lungs. The middle burner lies at the level of the solar plexus and affects your Stomach, Spleen, Liver and Gall Bladder. The lower burner lies at the level of the lower abdomen and affects your Small and Large Intestines, Kidneys and Bladder. These three burners of the body assist the transformative process of the Organs that lie within the various regions.

Although your Triple Burner has no physical Organ this doesn't mean that it has no physical symptoms – it is rather that its symptoms often overlap with those of the Organs it is associated with. When diagnosing you, your acupuncturist might check the temperature of each of these burners by placing a hand on each area. Palpation may indicate, for example, that you have a cold area in the chest or a very hot area in the solar plexus. Imbalance in the temperature of one area may indicate that the Triple Burner is imbalanced and is not transforming the Qi and Fluids in the Organs of that area. Alternatively one of the underlying Organs may be blocked or deficient.

MENTAL AND EMOTIONAL SIGNS AND SYMPTOMS

Treatment on the Triple Burner helps to create stability in the Fire Element and it can moderate any fluctuations in the stability of the Heart and the Heart Protector. It may also enable you to deal with 'non-intimate' contact, as opposed to the intimate contact associated with the Heart and Heart Protector.

How balanced are my Heart and Small Intestine and my Pericardium and Triple Burner?

1. Do you ever have circulatory problems such as cold hands and feet?
2. Do you ever feel your heart beating?
3. Do you ever feel anxious, restless, agitated and/or panicky?
4. Are you sometimes unable to find the right word or a wrong word comes out in place of the word you want?
5. Do you ever have insomnia, a poor memory or do you startle easily?
6. Do you ever have digestive symptoms such as abdominal pain, intestinal rumblings, diarrhoea or constipation?
7. Do you ever feel unclear in your head or find it difficult to clear your mind?
8. Do you ever feel vulnerable or easily hurt?

If the answer to at least three of the questions above is Yes, then you may have an imbalance in one or more of the Organs of the Fire Element – the Heart, Small Intestine, Pericardium or Triple Burner.

The Spleen and Stomach (Earth)

The Spleen – the transformer and transporter

> 'The Stomach and Spleen are responsible for storehouses and granaries. The five tastes stem from them.'
>
> *Su Wen*, Chapter 8

The Spleen and the Stomach work so closely together that they are the only paired Organs not mentioned separately in the *Su Wen*. Together they take responsibility for transforming all of the food and fluid in your body.

The Spleen Organ is very different from its Western counterpart and might be better translated as 'the digestive function'. This Organ oversees all transformation and transportation of food and fluid in the body.

PHYSICAL SIGNS AND SYMPTOMS

Once your food has been 'rotted and ripened' by the Stomach (more on that below), the Spleen's job is to take the pure essences from it and transform them into usable energy. This is then distributed to all the other Organs/Officials. Here it is refined to become the energy that feeds your body parts such as flesh, muscles, sense organs and even your thoughts (yes, thoughts need energy too!).

If the Spleen is strong, then the digestion is robust and a plentiful supply of Qi and Blood is created. In this case a person will have a good appetite, digestion, energy and muscle tone. If the Spleen is deficient a person may develop diarrhoea, a bloated abdomen, appetite disorders or low energy. The Spleen also transforms your Body Fluids. Spleen deficiency can cause them to accumulate, leading to oedema in the lower part of the body, Damp and Phlegm.

Along with its transformative function, the Spleen is also said to control the Blood. This means that it has a role in the formation of blood and that it also keeps the blood in your blood vessels. If the Spleen Qi is weak, your blood leaks out of the blood vessels and you may get bleeding symptoms. These include spotting between periods, blood in the stools, nosebleeds or bruising easily. Many chronic bleeding diseases can be treated through the Spleen.

The Spleen dominates your muscles and four limbs. The appearance of your muscles and the muscle tone indicates the relative strength of the Spleen. People with absorption problems due to a weak Spleen may find that food is not transformed into energy but into flesh and this can result in obesity or plumpness.

The mouth and lips, which are crucial in the process of eating and digestion, also reflect the condition of your Spleen. A healthy Spleen gives you a good sense of taste and healthy red lips. An unhealthy Spleen means you may become less sensitive to taste and your lips become paler. The Spleen Qi also enables your Organs to stay in place in your body – something Chinese medicine calls 'raising Qi'. Weakened Spleen Qi can lead to the Organs prolapsing and causing symptoms such as a prolapsed bowel, uterus or stomach, or even haemorrhoids. In this case, treating your Spleen can ensure the Organs return to their correct positions.

MENTAL AND EMOTIONAL SIGNS AND SYMPTOMS

As well as transforming food and fluids the Spleen also controls the quality of your thoughts. When your Spleen is functioning well you have clear intentions and the ability to turn your thoughts into actions. In this case you can think clearly, study diligently and gain satisfaction from small as well as larger achievements.

If your Spleen is imbalanced, you may be what is termed 'a worrier' or feel mentally unclear. Rather than being transformed, your thoughts may go round and round in your head without being assimilated. This may cause you to seem preoccupied or obsessed. Some people who have an imbalanced Spleen may find it difficult to complete or move on to new things. In this case they are unable to gain satisfaction and fulfilment and 'reap a harvest' from their achievements.

The Stomach – the controller of rotting and ripening

Chinese medicine poetically describes the job of the Stomach as one of 'rotting and ripening food and fluid'. This 'rotting and ripening' process takes place physically, mentally and emotionally.

PHYSICAL FUNCTIONS AND SIGNS AND SYMPTOMS

In Chinese medicine the 'Stomach' refers not only to the 'bag' that receives all of your food but also to the complete pathway of your food – the mouth where food enters, the oesophagus and the stomach itself. Chinese people freely admit to being obsessed by food. This is because they realise the important part it plays in keeping themselves healthy. Their greeting emphasises this. When Chinese people meet each other they don't say 'Hello, how are you?' Rather they say 'Have you eaten?' If your Stomach is strong it will propel the 'rotted and ripened' food downwards to the Small Intestine. If your Stomach is weak, food will stagnate there causing symptoms such as belching, vomiting, appetite disorders, stomach pains or aches, bloating or hiccups.

MENTAL AND EMOTIONAL SIGNS AND SYMPTOMS

Expressions like 'I can't stomach it' or 'It makes me want to heave' or 'I'm sick of it all' indicate that we understand that there is a close connection between the physical stomach and its emotional aspects. As well as rotting and ripening physically, your Stomach rots and ripens mentally. If your Stomach is strong it allows you to take in and digest information, ideas and thoughts so that you can use them in your everyday life. In this case, you can be nourished and gain satisfaction from what you do on a daily basis.

When your Stomach is weak it is unable to rot and ripen and you may have difficulty assimilating and getting nourished by what is around you. This may result in comfort eating and a pre-occupation with food. Alternatively, you may start to feel generally dissatisfied with the 'food' of your mind and emotions – your job, family or friends – because they do not nourish you. This can result in continually craving for more and never being quite content with what you already have.

How balanced are my Stomach and Spleen?

1. Do you ever have digestive disorders, for example diarrhoea, a bloating abdomen, a poor appetite, an appetite for unwholesome foods, belching or vomiting?
2. Do you have fluid problems such as oedema in the lower part of body, overweight and/or phlegm?
3. Do you sometimes have bleeding symptoms such as spotting between periods, blood in the stools, nosebleeds or bruising?
4. Are you less sensitive to taste than you would like to be?
5. Do you have a bearing-down sensation in your lower abdomen or have you ever had signs of a prolapse?
6. Are you a 'worrier' or do your thoughts sometimes go round and round in your head?
7. Do you comfort eat or often become unnecessarily preoccupied with food?

8. Do you often feel dissatisfied and unnourished by some of the things you do?

If the answer to at least three of the questions above is Yes, then you may have an imbalance in the Organs of the Earth Element – the Stomach and Spleen.

The Lungs and Large Intestine (Metal)

The Lungs – the receivers of Qi from the heavens

'The Lung holds the office of Minister and Chancellor.
The regulation of the life-giving network stems from it.'
Su Wen, Chapter 8

The Lungs are responsible for breathing. When they are healthy you breathe well and take in what in Chinese medicine is called 'heavenly Qi'. This Qi from the air you breathe mixes with the Qi from the Spleen to form the healthy Qi in your body.

PHYSICAL SIGNS AND SYMPTOMS

The movement and rhythm of the breath gives movement and rhythm to the whole of your body. If your respiration is even and regular, the healthy Qi moves smoothly throughout your body. When the Lungs are imbalanced, however, symptoms such as a cough, asthma or bronchitis can arise.

It is not only your breath that the Lungs propel and disperse into your body. The Lungs are also known as 'the upper source of Water'. They encourage the flow of water and fluids through your body, especially to the Kidneys, which are 'the lower source of Water'. If the fluids are not moved downwards to the

Kidneys, symptoms such as swelling of the face or urinary problems can arise.

The Lungs are also often described as the 'tender' or 'fragile' Organs. This is because, as the uppermost Organs in the body, they can easily be 'invaded' by pathogens, causing infections such as colds and influenza (see Chapter 9 for more on this and what is called an 'invasion of Wind'). If the Lungs are strong they ward off such infections and ensure that your immune system remains healthy. If you have weak Lungs you may have an increased susceptibility to all types of respiratory infections.

The tissues associated with the Lungs are the skin and hair. The skin, which is sometimes called the third Lung, reflects the state of your Lungs. For example, when you have a cold your hair will become lank and your skin dull. This indicates that your Lungs are temporarily weak. Many people with skin conditions also have some imbalance in their Lungs. When the Lungs are strong, your skin looks vibrant and your hair becomes glossy and shiny.

It is not surprising that the orifice connected with the Lungs is the nose, which has been called the 'thoroughfare for respiration'. It is through your nose that clear breath enters the Lungs and unclear is expelled. Many problems with the nose originate from weak Lungs. The throat is also affected by the Lungs and is said to be 'the door of the Lungs'. If your Lungs are weak you may have a weak voice or sometimes dislike speaking. Many nose and throat disorders, such as tonsillitis, sore throats, sinusitis and a blocked nose, may also be treated through the Lungs.

MENTAL AND EMOTIONAL SIGNS AND SYMPTOMS

The lungs take in the Qi from the 'heavens'. The Qi animates your body and mind giving you the ability to feel bodily sensation and enabling you to make a good connection with the world. If the Lungs are healthy, you will feel alive and vital and be able to take in information through your five senses – by seeing, feeling, hearing, smelling and tasting. They especially enable you to feel grief, which is the emotion associated with the Lungs. If your Lungs are not functioning well you may start to find that your senses are dulled and you are unable to feel physical sensation or emotion clearly. Grief is a feeling of emptiness or longing and if the lungs are weak you may feel cut off and alienated from people and the world and feel something is missing – but find that you can't put your finger on what it is.

In the section on physical signs and symptoms, I described how the Lungs protect you from infections and ensure that you have a healthy immune system. They also have a similar mental and emotional function and enable you to feel emotionally robust. If the Lungs are healthy you will be able to deal flexibly with and gain perspective on emotional situations. Weakened Lungs may cause you to feel fragile emotionally. This may lead you to react defensively if you feel criticised, and either show no emotion or have excessively strong emotions.

The Large Intestine – the drainer of the dregs

'The Large Intestine is responsible for transit.
The residue from transformation stems from it.'
Su Wen, Chapter 8

The Large Intestine has been given the title of the 'rubbish collector' or 'drainer of the dregs'. Its job is to eliminate all waste matter from the body. The job of rubbish collector is seen by some to be the lowliest job of all, but without good elimination you are unable to take anything in, not only physically but also mentally and emotionally. It is therefore an extremely important Organ.

PHYSICAL SIGNS AND SYMPTOMS

Most of your body's waste products are excreted through the bowel, via what Chinese medicine calls the 'descending' function of the Large Intestine. Some wastes are excreted through the skin, which is connected with the paired Organ, the Lungs. If the process of elimination is working well you have a regular bowel movement – once a day (often in the morning) and with a well-formed stool. Although there are obviously some variations in this regularity, any large deviation may indicate that the Large Intestine is not working as well as it might.

Problems with your Large Intestine can cause constipation, loose bowels, abdominal pain or other difficulties to do with elimination such as spots, blocked pores, and nose and throat disorders.

MENTAL AND EMOTIONAL SIGNS AND SYMPTOMS

A person whose Large Intestine is blocked mentally or emotionally may begin to feel 'mentally constipated' and be unable to let go of emotions and feelings. These emotions then start to build up and create 'psychological' waste matter in the form of resentment, guilt, pessimism or cynicism. The person may experience feeling increasingly cut off. The Lungs and Large Intestine are closely connected and together they can affect a person's ability both to take in (through the Lungs) and let go (through the Large Intestine). As the rubbish builds up a person may become increasingly negative in their thoughts and feelings. Treatment of the Large Intestine can enable the person to let go in order to move forward and change.

How balanced are my Lungs and Large Intestine?

1. Do you often have chest complaints such as a cough, asthma or bronchitis?
2. Do you easily catch colds and flu or have other infections such as sinusitis or tonsillitis?
3. Do you easily get spots, blocked pores or rashes or have poor-quality skin?
4. Do you sometimes feel unusually emotionally fragile and close off if you feel attacked?
5. Is your voice sometimes weak or do you sometimes dislike speaking?
6. Do you ever have bowel problems such as constipation or loose bowels or have abdominal pain or discomfort?
7. Do you ever have swelling of your face or any part of your face?
8. Do you ever feel 'mentally constipated' or easily overloaded?

If the answer to at least three of the questions above is Yes, then you may have an imbalance in the Organs of the Metal Element – the Lung and Large Intestine.

The Kidneys and Bladder (Water)

The Kidneys – the controller of fluid

> 'The Kidneys are responsible for the creation of power. Skill and ability stem from them.'
>
> *Su Wen*, Chapter 8

The Kidneys are responsible for ensuring that you have plentiful reserves of energy. They enable you to have enough physical, mental and emotional strength and determination. They are also the foundation of all water in the body and enable you to have fluid movements and sufficient moisture in your body.

PHYSICAL SIGNS AND SYMPTOMS

The Kidneys store the Essence which is the basis of your constitutional energy (see Chapter 6 for more on the Essence). To a large degree you inherit this Essence from your parents at conception. As a young child you have strong muscles and energy, fluid movements, moist skin and shiny hair. As you age your muscles grow weaker and you grow stiffer, your energy decreases, your skin wrinkles and your hair turns grey and starts to fall out. These are all signs that the moisture and strength of your Kidneys is diminishing. When this energy is finally exhausted, you die. In order to thrive your whole body depends on the Essence of the Kidneys. If the Kidney Essence becomes weakened early in your life, you will age prematurely.

The Kidneys are also in charge of ensuring that the underlying structures of the body remain strong and firm. The Essence is transformed into 'Marrow', which is the name given in Chinese medicine for the fluid that fills the brain and spinal cord,[3] and also bone and bone marrow. By 'filling' the brain it is said to give you the ability to be 'clever' and to think clearly. All bone development and repair depends on the Kidneys and the Marrow enables you to have a strong and healthy spine and bones. If a child's Marrow is weak, brittle or soft bones may result. In an adult weak Marrow may result in weak legs, a stiff spine or osteoporosis. Teeth are also an offshoot of the Kidneys and the ears their orifice. If your Kidneys are weak your teeth will not be strong and your hearing will diminish.

The Kidneys lie in the lower body and give strength and vitality to the lower back and lower abdomen. Many fertility problems, backaches, knee and urinary problems can result from Kidney weakness.

Finally, the Kidneys 'control the reception of Qi'. After you have taken a breath of air into your Lungs, the Kidneys 'grasp' it, thus allowing the breath to deepen. The Lungs are not the only cause of breathing problems. Chinese medicine teaches that many conditions such as asthma, coughs and shallow breathing can also be caused by Kidney disharmonies.

MENTAL AND EMOTIONAL SIGNS AND SYMPTOMS

Chinese medicine teaches that Kidneys house the will. If you have strong Kidneys you are likely to have the drive to press forward to fulfil your potential in life as well as the will to survive and continue the species. There are two sides to the will. The Yang side is a forceful part of you that gives you the power to make fundamental changes and shifts in your life. The Yin side is deeper and more subtle. It is more about the small, steady, inevitable changes that go on in you internally as you pass through the different stages of growth and development in your life. If your Kidneys are weak you may lack the drive to meet life's challenges or overly compensate with a very strong will.

As you grow older your will should be transformed into wisdom. Wise people recognise that they can deal with some things in life and not others.[4] Although the passage of time weakens the physical aspects of the Essence and Kidney Qi, this spiritual dimension should mature and strengthen.

The Bladder – the controller of storage of fluids

'The Bladder is responsible for the regions and cities.
It stores the Body Fluids. The transformation of Qi then gives out their power.'

Su Wen, Chapter 8

The function of the Bladder is to control the distribution of fluids and it has the longest pathway in the whole body. It is closely linked to the Kidneys and at times it may be difficult to distinguish the functions of these two Organs.

PHYSICAL FUNCTIONS AND SIGNS AND SYMPTOMS

The Bladder's job is a simple one. It receives the fluids from the Kidneys, transforms any remaining pure fluids and then stores them until they are excreted. When the Bladder is obstructed this may cause symptoms such as cystitis, burning or difficulty urinating. A deficient Bladder may cause incontinence, bed-wetting and other urinary problems.

The Bladder pathway travels from the foot, up the back and over the neck and head to end at the corner of the eye. Many conditions such as backaches, headaches and sciatica can be caused by an imbalance along this channel.

MENTAL AND EMOTIONAL SIGNS AND SYMPTOMS

When the Bladder is weakened you may feel drained and under strain, both mentally and emotionally. Your mental fluidity may seem to dry up and this can affect the flow of your thoughts, causing them to seem jerky. It may be difficult to move your mind from subject to subject. This may happen, for instance, when someone is overcome with anxiety when speaking in public. The drying up may also cause you to become more cautious and careful. Rather than seeing the big picture you may see only a small part of what is possible for you to achieve.

How balanced are my Kidneys and Bladder?

1. Do you sometimes have insufficient reserves of energy, or do you have to be careful not to overdo it?
2. Do you have a stiff spine, weak bones or poor teeth?

3. Do you get back problems or feel cold in your lower back?

4a. (For women only.) Have you ever had difficulty conceiving or do you have insufficient blood when you menstruate?

4b. (For men only.) Have you ever been told you have a low sperm count?

5. Do you ever feel unable to breathe in deeply?

6. Do you sometimes feel driven and/or sometimes feel completely lacking in any drive?

7. Do you ever have the urge to get up in the night to urinate?

8. Do you ever feel jerky in your speech or the flow of your thoughts?

If the answer to at least three of the questions above is Yes, then you may have an imbalance in the Organs of the Water Element – the Kidneys and Bladder.

Summary of the functions of the Yin Organs

Yin Organ	Liver	Heart and Pericardium	Spleen	Lung	Kidney
Main function	Ensures the smooth flow of Qi. Stores Blood	Moves the Blood. Controls the Blood vessels	Oversees transformation and transportation. Controls the Blood	Creates Qi and facilitates breathing. Descends and disperses Qi	Stores essence. Controls the reception of Qi

Summary of the functions of the Yang organs

Yang Organ	Gall Bladder	Small Intestine and Triple Burner	Stomach	Large Intestine	Bladder
Main function	Stores and excretes bile. Enables good decision making	Separates pure from impure	Rots and ripens food and drink	Receives food and drink from the Small Intestine and excretes the waste	Transforms and excretes water

The Five Elements and the Organs

The Five Elements are a fundamental part of Chinese Medicine theory which teaches that each pair of the Organs discussed on page 153 is represented by one of Five Elements[5] (there are twelve Organs and the Fire Element is associated with Four Organs). The Chinese character for an Element is '*xing*'. This depicts something that is a moving force, a phase, or something transforming or changing. Chinese Medicine teaches that our health is a harmonious balance of the Qi found in all of the qualities of the Elements.

The names of the Five Elements poetically describe five qualities found in nature, they are: Wood, Fire, Earth, Metal and Water. As well as being associated with the Organs, these Elements are also associated with many other qualities including a season, a climate, a taste, a colour, a voice tone, an emotion and an odour.

The *Sheng* and *Ke* Cycles

The Five Elements all relate to each other and are often depicted as flowing in a clockwise direction from one to the other. One Element feeds the next. For example, Water feeds Wood, Wood feeds Fire, Fire feeds Earth, and so on (see diagram on page 156). This is called the *sheng* or generating cycle. Each Element also is tempered by the others, via the *ke* or controlling cycle.

Some Important Five Element associations

	Wood	Fire	Earth	Metal	Water
Colour	Blue-Green	Red	Yellow	White	Blue-Black
Voice tone	Shout	Laugh	Sing	Weep	Groan
Emotion	Anger	Joy	Worry/ Sympathy	Grief	Fear
Odour	Rancid	Scorched	Fragrant	Rotten	Putrid
Sense organ	Eye	Tongue	Mouth and lips	Nose	Ear
Generates	Nails	Complexion	Fat	Body hair	Teeth
Tissue or body part	Tendons and ligaments	Blood and blood vessels	Muscles and flesh	Skin and nose	Bones and bone marrow
Season	Spring	Summer	Late Summer	Autumn	Winter
Climate	Wind	Heat	Damp	Dryness	Cold
Taste	Sour	Bitter	Sweet	Pungent	Salty
Yin Organ	Liver	Heart/ Pericardium	Spleen	Lungs	Kidney
Yang Organ	Gall Bladder	Small Intestine/ Triple Burner	Stomach	Large Intestine	Bladder

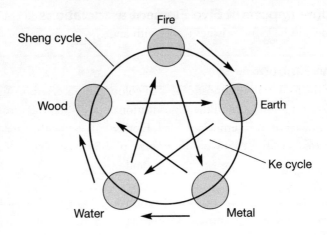

What is a Constitutional Imbalance?

Chinese medicine teaches that everyone is born with one of the Five Elements slightly weaker than the others and this is known as the 'Constitutional Factor'.[6] Because all the Elements and therefore the Organs are linked, the one that was originally imbalanced gradually affects all the others, rather like a weak link in a chain. The weakness of the Constitutional Element creates many different signs and symptoms which can be detected in our facial colour, voice tone, odour and emotional state.

If one Element is imbalanced it will have an important effect on your personality and behaviour as well as your physical health. For example, if you have a Constitutional Factor in the Earth Element affecting your Stomach and Spleen Organs, you might have a tinge of yellow in your facial colour, a singing quality in your voice tone, an odour that is slightly fragrant and a tendency to worry or be overly sympathetic. On the other hand, a person who has a Constitutional Factor in the Wood Element and the Liver and Gall Bladder Organs is more likely to have a greenish facial colour, a more strident or clipped voice tone and have more issues to do with anger.

The Emotion

Of the four main diagnostic areas of colour, sound, emotion and odour, an imbalance in the Constitutional Factor has the greatest impact on your emotions. Each Element gives you the capacity to feel an area of emotion in a positive way and when weakened, you struggle to feel this and instead have more negative experiences.

In the context of the constitutional imbalance 'emotion' means a habitual feeling state rather than a fleeting one-off feeling. Having issues around an emotion or even being an angry or a fearful person is very different from temporarily feeling angry or fearful then dealing with the emotion and returning to 'normal'. The imbalance in the Element and therefore the emotion leads to the manifestation of certain behavioural characteristics as well as the signs and symptoms associated with the Organs discussed earlier in this chapter.

Treating your constitution

Diagnosis of your Constitutional Factor

In order to diagnose your Constitutional imbalance an acupuncturist will read your colour, voice tone, emotion and odour. An assessment of the other characteristics of the Elements and Organs is then used to back this up. A diagnosis of your Constitutional Factor is formed from these observations.

Confirming your Constitutional Factor

Confirmation of the Constitutional Factor comes when you have treatment. To treat your Constitutional Factor, your acupuncturist uses points along the channels corresponding to the Element of your Constitutional Factor. For example, if you have a Constitutional Factor in the Wood Element your acupuncturist will pick points from the Liver and Gall Bladder channels, and someone with a Constitutional Factor in the Earth Element will be treated using points from the Stomach and Spleen channels. Provided no obstructions or blocks are present you are likely to feel an enhanced sense of well-being either immediately after treatment or, cumulatively, after a few treatments.

This sense of enhanced well-being comes about from being treated at the root cause of your problem. As well as feeling better, many of your symptoms will also go away over a longer period of time. Other signs, such as the harmonising of your pulses, also indicates a change in your Constitutional Element. Signs and symptoms that do not change from treating the Constitutional Factor can then be dealt with by treating other Organs, substances such as *qi*, Blood, Body Fluids, essence and *shen* or pathogens such as Wind, Cold, Damp, Dryness or Heat.

Summary

- Chinese medicine teaches that there are twelve Organs, which are divided into six Yang Organs and six Yin Organs.
- It emphasises an Organ's wider energetic functions which have physical as well as a mental and emotional signs and symptoms.
- The twelve Organs are paired together as the Liver and Gall Bladder, Heart and Small Intestine, Pericardium and Triple Burner, Stomach and Spleen, Lung and Large Intestine, and Kidney and Bladder.

- Each pair of Organs is associated with one of Five Elements which are Wood, Fire, Earth, Metal and Water.
- One effective way of treating the cause of your illness is to treat the Organs and Elements of your Constitutional Factor.
- Treatment on the Constitutional Factor can help you to feel enhanced well-being. This comes from being treated at the root cause of your problem.

8

How Your Acupuncturist Forms a Diagnosis

The importance of a diagnosis

If you've been filling in the questionnaires throughout the book you will now have some information about the balance of your health in a number of areas:[1]

- whether a **pathogen** such as Wind, Cold, Damp, Heat or Dryness is affecting your system
- whether your **emotions** are affecting your health
- whether you are more **Yin** or **Yang**
- whether one of the **Substances** of Qi, Essence, Blood, Body Fluids and Shen is out of balance
- which of your **Organs** is most imbalanced and which Element might be your **Constitutional Factor**.

When you come for treatment your acupuncturist will consider all of the areas above by asking you many detailed questions. She or he will also make some important observations about your pulse, your tongue, the colour of your face, the balance of your emotions and your voice tone. Your practitioner will then put these together to create a complete picture of your health. The balance of your Yin and Yang, the substances, the Organs and your Constitutional Factor are never considered in isolation and your practitioner will synthesise this information to make a complete and holistic diagnosis.

Early on in Chapter 3, I briefly introduced you to the initial diagnosis session that is carried out when you first come for treatment. In this chapter I'll discuss the questions you might be asked and how your practitioner uses this information to decide which treatment will bring you to a healthy balance.

Coming for a diagnosis

Why carry out a diagnosis?

A full diagnosis ensures that you are given individual and correct treatment. An acupuncturist understands that health is a very positive state that doesn't just involve a reduction of your symptoms. As a result of treatment, as well as a change in your physical health, your spirits might improve. You might have more vitality and energy and feel calmer or more contented with life. Because you are unique, two people with the same symptoms will not have the same diagnosis and will therefore have different treatment.

When you read about the functions of the Organs in Chapter 7, you might have realised that most symptoms can come from a number of different causes. Take, for example, a common symptom such as tiredness. This can be caused by deficiency in the Spleen, Kidney, Lung or Heart Qi. It can also arise because the Qi is stagnant, making a person feel weary and de-motivated. Damp or Phlegm can cause tiredness which makes a person feel heavy and lethargic. Finally, Blood deficiency causes yet another type of tiredness, making you feel weak and insubstantial.

Headaches are another example. Chinese medicine teaches that these can be caused by an imbalance in the Liver, Gall Bladder, Stomach or Kidneys as well as by either deficient or full Qi, Blood, Yin or Yang.

You'll notice from the above examples that when making a diagnosis your acupuncturist is aware of interactions between your Yin and Yang, your substances and your Organs. She or he also bears in mind your underlying constitutional imbalance. Together these are synthesised into a whole diagnosis.

What your practitioner needs to know in order to make a diagnosis

The diagnosis is both verbal and non-verbal and your acupuncturist will be noticing many things about you. Your voice tone, your posture and your facial expressions all contribute to the diagnosis. There are four main strands to the diagnosis, which are called 'to hear', 'to ask', 'to see' and 'to feel'.

Why does my practitioner ask these questions?

Below are the kinds of questions and observations that your acupuncturist will make. Although many of them appear to have nothing to do with your main complaint, they give your practitioner a complete picture of your health. Without this picture, it may be impossible to understand the root cause underlying your signs and symptoms. Sometimes your acupuncturist will ask you all of these questions and at other times she or he will follow 'leads' and ask specific questions that prove or disprove the proposed diagnosis. If you have an acute condition, or are in pain, she or he will often treat your condition first, then ask more questions to ascertain the underlying problem later on.

To ask and to hear

Getting to know you

When you first come for treatment, your acupuncturist will often just chat for a short while. She or he will want to know something about you – this could be your work, hobbies and interests. This is partly because of a genuine interest in finding out more about you. It's also because she or he knows that good rapport helps you to feel comfortable about being treated. This is especially important during the diagnosis, when you can tell your acupuncturist about areas of your life that have affected your health in the past or now.

The main complaint

One of the first questions you are likely to be asked is about your main complaint and why you have come to be treated. Although acupuncture aims to treat you as a whole, everyone usually has at least one, if not two or more particular reasons for coming to treatment. You don't have to have a main complaint as your acupuncturist can give you preventative treatment in order to keep you well. Most commonly, however, people come for treatment with a physical, mental or emotional problem.

Below are some of the questions you may be asked about your main complaint:

- What problem brings you to treatment?
- When did it start, and did you notice anything happening at that time to cause it?
- Where is your problem located?
- If you have pain or a sensation, what is it like? For example, it could be heavy, throbbing, gripping or numb. It could also be dull or strong, continuous or intermittent.
- What makes your complaint better or worse?

- What does the complaint prevent you from doing?
- Do you have any other accompanying symptoms?
- What other treatments have you had for it? (Other therapies, medications, etc.)

Because your symptoms manifest individually, your practitioner will want to know as many details as possible about them and how they affect you.

Other questions your practitioner might ask

Having found out the initial information about your main complaint, your practitioner will then ask about many of your bodily systems. Although some of these questions may not appear to be connected to your main complaint they are still important as they give the practitioner a full picture of you and your health.

Sleep. How you sleep reflects the functioning of many of your Organs, especially your Heart, Heart Protector, Kidneys and Liver. You might be asked about when you go to bed and when you rise, whether you fall asleep easily, how deeply you sleep, if you dream and whether you wake in the night. If you do wake you might be asked why you wake. For instance, is it due to pain or anxiety, because you need to pass urine, or does there seem to be no reason at all?

Appetite, food and taste. Many people say that their appetite is 'too good'! This often means that they feel they eat too much or snack a lot and, like many of us, they are conscious of their weight. Weight problems are often due to imbalances in your digestive Organs such as your Stomach, Spleen, Liver, Gall Bladder and Intestines. What you eat also has a profound effect on your energy. You may be asked how well you digest your food, what you eat on a 'normal' day, when you eat, whether you have any discomfort after eating and the pattern of your bowel movements.

You may be asked about your taste preferences, as this can reflect the functioning of many of your Organs. For example, people with a desire for salty food may have an imbalance in the Kidneys, while those who like a sour taste may have Liver problems. The taste connected with the Spleen is sweet. This is the subtle sweetness of carrots, rice or many fruits, rather than the strong sweetness of sugar. Too much sugary food can deplete the Spleen and lead to further craving for the sweet taste.

Thirst and drink. Your practitioner will want to know about your fluid intake generally. This can reveal information about your Kidneys, Bladder and Stomach as well as your Body Fluids. You may also be asked about whether you prefer hot or cold drinks, as this can reflect the amount of heat or cold in your system.

Urination. You may be asked about how often you pass urine, the colour of your urine and if you ever have urgency to pass water. This will give your practitioner information about your Body Fluids and the functioning of your Kidneys and Bladder as well as your Lungs.

Perspiration. How much you perspire and when you perspire can reflect fullness or deficiency of Yin or Yang as well as the functioning of many of your Organs including the Heart, Lungs and Kidneys.

Women's health. Gynaecology is a huge subject in Chinese medicine. I have seen acupuncture benefit many women who have come with a range of conditions including menstrual and pre-menstrual problems, fertility problems, conditions arising during pregnancy and childbirth and problems related to the menopause and discharges.[2] Your practitioner is likely to ask for information about the history of your periods and current menstrual patterns, as well as many other specific questions. This will give feedback about the functioning of many Organs including your Liver, Kidneys, Heart and Spleen, as well as your Qi, Essence, Blood, Body Fluids and Shen and the balance of your Yin and Yang.

Head, Body, Ears and Eyes. Your practitioner will want to check how every part of your body is functioning, from the top of your head to your toes. To do this she or he will ask you questions aimed at finding out about the functioning of each area. These might include questions such as, 'Do you ever have any headaches?' 'How are your eyes?' 'How is your hearing?' 'Do you have aches and pains in any joints?' or 'Do you ever have backache?' If you say yes, you will then be asked more specific questions about that area. For example, headaches and migraines, like other symptoms, manifest in many different ways and have many potential causes. Your acupuncturist will want to know if they are arising from an imbalance in your Liver – the most common cause – or another Organ.

Heat or cold preferences. Your temperature preferences provide important information about the fullness or deficiency of your Yin and Yang. For example, if you feel the cold, this may reveal that you don't have enough Yang energy to warm you up and your cooling Yin energy is correspondingly too strong. On the other hand, if you often feel hot, this may indicate that you are somewhat deficient in cooling Yin energy and correspondingly have too much warming Yang energy. Heat or Cold can get stuck in the body. For example, many fertility problems are caused by Cold in the uterus and Heat can cause many headaches.

Season and climate. People can be affected positively or negatively during different seasons. For example, some people love the stillness of autumn while others find it makes them feel melancholic. Others experience certain symptoms at different times of year. For instance, they may feel depressed in the winter, find themselves beset by colds in the springtime or suffer skin rashes during the summer months. Sometimes the climate has a profound effect on people's symptoms. For example, Wind or Damp can make someone's joint pains or headaches substantially better or worse. (For more about climate and your health see Chapter 5.)

Time of day. In Chapter 4 I briefly described a two-hour period when each Organ has a greater amount of Qi passing through it. Patients sometimes notice that they feel better or worse at certain times and this can indicate the health of the corresponding Organs. For example, people who frequently wake up in the early hours between 1 am and 3 am may have an imbalanced Liver. If they also lie awake thinking and making plans this would further support the diagnosis. The time of maximum Qi for the Kidneys is between 5 pm and 7 pm. If people become particularly tired at this time, but later recover their energy, this may be indicative of an imbalance in their Kidneys. The time of maximum Qi for the Large Intestine is from 5 am to 7 am. People who regularly open their bowels first thing in the morning often have a well-functioning intestinal system. If they then enjoy a hearty breakfast between 7 am and 9 am this may indicate a well-functioning Stomach and at the same time help to keep the Stomach healthy, as it is 'Stomach' time and the most beneficial time to eat.

Personal history. A famous Chinese doctor who lived in New York put great emphasis on different phases in your life and how they can affect you. He said that some crucial times in relation to your overall health are puberty, setting up home with a partner, childbirth and menopause. These are times when you are changing physically, mentally and emotionally. Some patients say things like, 'I've never been the same since puberty' or 'I first became ill at the time of my menopause.' Others observe that 'I really blossomed when I had my children' or 'after I got married my health changed for the better'. The acupuncturist needs to know about your history in order to assess these and other factors to do with your overall health now.

Family history. Your acupuncturist will usually want to know about your parents' health and if there are any illnesses which tend to run in the family. This will give her or him a clue as to whether there is any inherited basis to your complaint.

Medical history. Whenever a symptom arises in any of the above areas, your acupuncturist will probably ask you for more information about the history of that symptom. In order to have a fuller picture of you, she or he is also likely to ask you about your medical history. This helps to ascertain whether your problems began before birth, during your childhood or later on in adulthood. Many people have a number of different ailments and these have often begun during different periods.

Current lifestyle. You will be asked about your current lifestyle and areas such as your diet, work, rest, and leisure activities. This helps your practitioner to understand how your current lifestyle is affecting your health.

Medications. Your practitioner will want to know all the details about any medication you are taking. She or he will not expect you to cut down or stop taking any prescribed drugs. If and when you wish to reduce the dosage of any medication, your practitioner will want to work with your doctor to ensure that you cut down safely.

Ancient Chinese doctors – *Bian Que* and his diagnostic skills

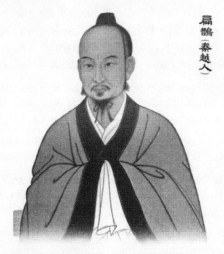

Bian Que (pronounced 'Bee-an Chur') lived around 200 BC. He was said to have been the most eminent diagnostician in China in his time and many legends arose about him. His fame spread after he was called upon to treat an ailing prince. By the time he arrived at the royal palace he was told that the prince had died and was being prepared for his funeral. On seeing the 'dead' prince, *Bian Que* realised that he was merely in a coma and successfully revived him using acupuncture and herbs. His father, the king, was eternally grateful and the doctor's reputation was assured. He was subsequently hailed as having the ability to see inside his patients and to diagnose how each internal organ was functioning!

A famous acupuncture book called the *Nan Jing* or Classic of Difficulties was attributed to *Bian Que*. It probably wasn't actually written by him but may have been a distillation of the theories he formed during his medical practice.

To see and other observations

While your acupuncturist is asking you questions she or he will also be making observations. These include your facial colour, voice tone and emotions as well as your habitual postures, gestures and facial expression. She or he will also ask to see your tongue. This non-verbal diagnosis is as useful to the practitioner as asking questions.

Colour. When an Element or Organ becomes imbalanced this may show in the colour on your face. If the Wood Element is obstructed, for example, this may manifest as a green colour; if your Fire Element is weak, you may look pale. A deficient Earth Element may create a slight yellow hue and if you have an imbalanced Water Element you may look dark under the eyes. These colours will change as treatment progresses. The colours are best seen beside the eye but can also be seen around the mouth and under the eye.

Sound. Voice tone changes according to what you are talking about. It is normal, for instance, to have a shouting voice when you are angry, or a laughing voice if you are happy about something. Sometimes a voice tone will be inappropriate to what a person is saying. For example, if a person shouts out words of sympathy, groans when talking about happy times or has a weeping tone when angry this may reflect an energetic imbalance in one of the associated Elements.

Odour. As well as using their eyes and ears, your acupuncturist also will use their sense of smell. Each of us has our own characteristic body odour. When you were a child you may have noticed this more, especially when you had close physical contact with people.

As people's energy becomes less balanced, their odour will change. If, for example, you become overheated or your Heart energy becomes imbalanced, you may start to exude a slightly scorched odour, while a malfunctioning Spleen or Earth Element can cause you to have a sweeter smell. If your acupuncturist detects these odours it provides important diagnostic information that can be monitored as you change.

Emotion. Your acupuncturist may also observe your emotional expression. When you are ill the expression of your feelings can become imbalanced. Some people become more irritable, others find that they can no longer laugh as they used to and others become more anxious or fearful. By observing and understanding these emotions, your acupuncturist can pinpoint where your imbalance lies and what treatment you need. As patients become healthier their emotions often become more stable. Sometimes patients don't realise that they have felt 'out of sorts', but report after a few treatments, 'I feel better in myself.'

Diagnosis of your colour, sound, emotion and odour is especially useful when your practitioner diagnoses your constitutional imbalance.

Posture and gestures. Body language and posture can be important. For example, if your Lung or Heart Qi is imbalanced this may be reflected in an underdeveloped chest area. Patients with Damp may have slightly heavy legs if they are women or paunches if they are men. The Kidney Qi affects the spine. When people feel full of vitality they can stand up straight. As the Qi becomes deficient people can no longer hold themselves upright. It is noticeable that people who are less stressed have a more erect posture than people who are overworked and have worn out their Kidneys.

Facial expression. An acupuncturist learns to read your facial expression. This enables her or him to understand your emotions. For example, Chinese medicine calls two vertical lines on the forehead 'Liver lines'. These are caused by constant feelings of frustration and stress, which ultimately affect the

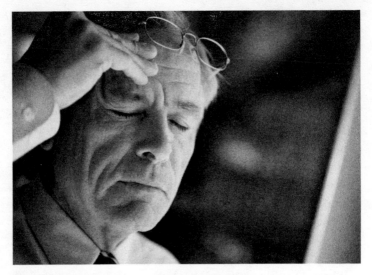

An example of a face with 'Liver lines'

Liver. Another example is the obicularis oculi muscle that surrounds the eye.[3] It is only activated if a person is truly smiling. If a person is pretending to smile, it will not move. This may indicate an imbalance in a person's joy and the Fire Element. The eyes themselves are the best indicators of someone's emotional state. They are 'the windows of the soul', and reflect the state of your mind-spirit as well as any of your emotions.

The mind-spirit. In order to assess your mind-spirit, your acupuncturist will observe characteristics such as the sparkle in your eyes and the clarity of your communication. It may be necessary to use points that treat the spirit so that a person can return to their full level of health and vitality.

Tongue diagnosis

The colour, shape, moisture, movement, coating and areas of your tongue are used to diagnose the state of your internal organs. Disharmony often shows on the tongue before any signs and symptoms have manifested. In fact, it is one of the few places where you can see the state of your internal Organs on the outside of your body. A healthy tongue is pale red in colour, fairly moist, fits snugly into the mouth and has a thin white coating. Your practitioner will be observing signs on the tongue that include its colour, shape, 'areas', spots, cracks, movement, moisture and coating. Below are some of the most common observations that your practitioner will make.

Colour. If your tongue looks redder than normal, this shows the presence of Heat. A pale tongue indicates Cold as well as Blood deficiency. Because the tongue is filled with Blood, it will naturally become paler when Blood is deficient. A purple tongue usually indicates stagnation within the body.

Shape. A tongue can become swollen and may have tooth marks around the edge. This is often due to excess Body Fluids, for example Damp being stuck in the body, or the Yang energy becoming deficient so that the body becomes cold and Body Fluids don't move. A thin tongue body can mean a lack of Body Fluids.

Areas. Each area corresponds to different Organs in the body. (See the diagram on page 37.) An area can be wet or dry, thin or swollen, pale or red according to which Organ of the body is out of balance. For instance, red sides to the tongue can mean Heat in the Liver and Gall Bladder, red in the centre can mean Heat in the Stomach and red at the tongue tip can mean Heat in the Heart. Sometimes the tongue has red 'spots' at the tip, indicating a tendency to become easily emotionally upset.

Cracks. Cracks indicate that the Yin Qi that should be creating moisture is becoming deficient. A crack in the centre of the tongue can indicate Stomach Yin deficiency. Cracks travelling to the tip will point to Heart Yin deficiency. A crack in the midline with small cracks coming from it often shows Kidney Yin deficiency.

Coating. A normal tongue coating is thin and white. Changes in the thickness of this 'fur' can indicate the fullness or deficiency of your condition. The tongue coating can sometimes change quite rapidly. For example, when you have an infection, you might notice that your tongue coating is thicker than normal and you might keep cleaning your teeth to clear it. As soon as this infection is over, it usually disappears. A Damp or Phlegm condition can also cause the coating to become thicker, but this is usually longer term. If you are Dry and Yin deficient your tongue coating can become thinner than normal and may even peel in some places. The colour of your coating indicates Heat or Cold: a white coating indicates Cold and a yellow coating more Heat.

Which tongue am I?

Thin white coating
Pale red body
Moist

A Normal Tongue

Thin white sticky coating
Teeth marks
Pale
Wet

QI Deficiency
Leading to Damp

Thin
Pale
Dry

Blood Deficiency

Red
Cracks
Little or no coating
Dry

Yin Deficiency

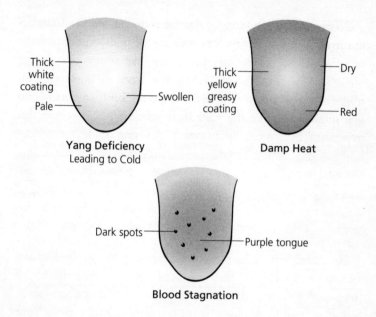

Thick white coating

Pale

Swollen

Yang Deficiency
Leading to Cold

Thick yellow greasy coating

Dry

Red

Damp Heat

Dark spots

Purple tongue

Blood Stagnation

To feel

This aspect of your diagnosis includes taking your pulses, feeling areas of your structure such as your joints and spine, and examining other aspects such as your nails and skin, as well as feeling the temperature on your torso.

Pulse diagnosis

Pulse-taking is both an art and a science and it forms a very important part of diagnosis and treatment. It is completely different from the pulse-taking carried out by conventional doctors and nurses who are feeling your pulse rate only. Your acupuncturist feels your pulses on the radial artery of both wrists. Reading the pulses enables her or him to gain information about your Qi as well as the state of your Organs. Each pulse position is associated with different Organs, as shown on the diagram below.

Pulse positions and Organs

	Left arm	Right arm
Distal (closest to the extremity)	Small Intestine/Heart	Lung/Large Intestine
Middle	Gall Bladder/Liver	Spleen/Stomach
Proximal (furthest from the extremity)	Bladder/Kidney	Pericardium/Triple Burner

The pulses reflect the internal functioning of your body, mind and spirit. Sometimes they are very deep down, indicating a deep-seated disease; at other times very near the surface, which can show that a condition is on the outside of the body. Your pulses might also be strong or weak, indicating the strength of your Qi, or too taut or 'wiry' because the Qi is blocked or you feel tense.

There are 15 basic qualities and 28 main pulse qualities that your acupuncturist might feel. These qualities vary according to the depth, width, strength, shape, rhythm and rate of the pulse. A normal pulse is well rounded, not too strong or weak, narrow or wide, fast or slow or superficial or deep in its position.

Even the healthiest people don't necessarily have 'normal' pulses. Your pulses express your individuality and change according to how you are feeling, the seasons and to some extent the time of day. The pulses also alter during an acupuncture treatment, indicating whether you have had enough treatment or if more is required.[4]

Some common pulse qualities and their meanings

Deficient. This pulse has no strength and indicates that the Qi is weak.

Full. This is a pounding, full and hard pulse that indicates a full condition or obstruction to the Qi.

Floating. This pulse is felt close to the surface of the body and often indicates that there is an invasion of Wind-Cold or Heat close to the exterior of the body.

Deep. This can only be felt with heavier pressure on the wrist and indicates disharmony deeper within the body.

Thin. The width of this pulse is thinner than normal. It often indicates that the Blood is deficient.

Slippery. This pulse feels as if it slips away from the finger. This quality often indicates the presence of Damp or Phlegm and it can also be felt in pregnancy.

Wiry. This pulse feels as if it is stretched tight like a wire or guitar string. It indicates that the Liver Qi is stagnant or that a person is in pain.

Choppy. This pulse feels a bit like a 'choppy sea'. It indicates there is disharmony in the Blood, which may be deficient or stagnant.

Structure

If you have treatment for a painful condition such as a shoulder pain, backache or stomach pains, your acupuncturist will want to examine the area. She or he will palpate the area carefully and by doing so find out how severe the pain is. Dull pain is often caused by deficient Qi, while severe pain commonly arises from an excess condition such as Wind, Cold or Damp. If the pain is in your joints your acupuncturist will find out whether your movement is restricted or not and whether your joints are more hot or cold. This is important information both diagnostically and because it will change to reflect progress during treatment.

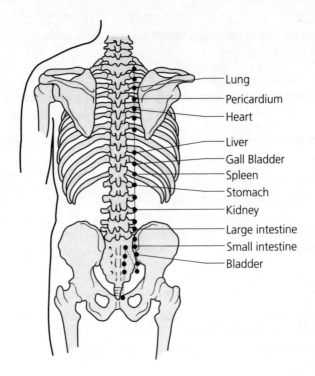

Lung
Pericardium
Heart
Liver
Gall Bladder
Spleen
Stomach
Kidney
Large intestine
Small intestine
Bladder

Touch

Your practitioner will examine your skin and nails. Problems with the nails are often caused by Liver conditions and especially indicate that the Liver has deficient Blood. Dry skin can have many causes, such as drying up from Yin deficiency, failure of the Lung Qi to moisturise the skin or lack of nourishment from the Blood. Greasy skin can often indicate that someone has Damp in their system.

Your practitioner might feel the temperature of different areas of your torso to tell whether the underlying organs are working well. She or he might also feel for tightness in areas along the spine or press on certain points that may be sensitive. If a point by the outside of the knee is tender, for instance, it could indicate that you have an inflamed gall bladder or gallstones. Tender points along the spine, as shown in the diagram, are associated with the corresponding Organs being out of balance.

'Red flag' areas

Your acupuncturist's training gives her or him a substantial knowledge of conventional medicine as well as Chinese medicine. She or he has been taught to notice any warning feature that could indicate that you may have a serious condition that requires diagnosis and treatment by a Western practitioner. If necessary your practitioner will refer you to a qualified medical doctor.

Putting it together – how the acupuncturist thinks of you

Having finished asking you questions and making observations your practitioner will sift through this information and pull it together to form a diagnosis. When making the diagnosis she or he decides which of your Organs are constitutionally weak and which have been affected by later events, such as emotional traumas, climatic conditions or lifestyle. Your practitioner also decides on the balance of your Yin and Yang and the interaction of the Substances with the Elements, Organs and channels. Having sorted through this information she or he decides how best to treat you.

To demonstrate how the diagnosis fits together we'll now look at one of the patients who was discussed in Chapter 2 and find out more about her diagnosis.

Case history – Josie

JOSIE'S PROBLEMS

You may remember that Josie came for treatment for fertility problems. She had two children but had been unable to conceive a third. About three months after she started treatment her mother died suddenly and she was devastated. For some months the emphasis of treatment shifted to helping her through this difficult time. When she felt ready, she tried to conceive again and a few months later she succeeded. She now has a seven–year–old child. She continues to have preventative treatment in order to remain well.

JOSIE'S DIAGNOSIS AND TREATMENT

Josie's Constitutional Factor was in her Water Element. Her facial colour was blue, especially beside her eyes, her voice tone was groaning and she often felt extremely fearful for no obvious reason. For example, when she first came for treatment she had 'catastrophic fantasies' that her husband might have a fatal car accident and she feared for his life whenever he went out. After a few treatments she said that she still had the fantasies but was not worried by them. Now she doesn't have them at all.

The Kidneys, the main Organ associated with her Water Element, were also out of balance. She had no warming Yang energy in her lower abdomen, causing this area to be Cold. The Coldness caused her infertility. Treating the Yang of her Kidneys and directly warming her lower abdomen with moxibustion helped her infertility, and her general energy and well-being too.

As well as her constitutional Water imbalance, she had some Dampness which caused her to hold water and to feel heavy in her limbs. This was treated via points on her Spleen. She also initially had some Liver Qi stagnation which caused premenstrual tension. This was helped by specific treatment carried out prior to her period. She no longer has any pre-menstrual problems at all.

Finally, the death of her mother literally broke her Heart. During the time that she was so traumatised much of her treatment was focused on strengthening her Heart. This enabled her gradually to come to terms with her loss and over time she gradually felt more peaceful inside.

She now comes for treatment about every six to eight weeks and the main treatment principle is to support her Bladder and Kidney function. If other imbalances start to arise I support these, thus keeping her energy in a healthy balance and enabling her to remain well.

Summary

- When your practitioner carries out a diagnosis, all of the information and observation she or he gathers is put together in order to make a complete and holistic diagnosis of you.
- There are four main strands to the diagnosis: 'to hear', 'to ask', 'to see' and 'to feel'.
- You will be questioned about your main complaint, as well as areas such as your sleep, appetite and perspiration, and also your past history, personal history and family history. This constitutes the 'to hear' and 'to ask' part of the diagnosis.
- The observation and other aspects of 'to see' includes observation of your facial colour, voice tone, odour and emotions as well as habitual postures, gestures, facial expression and tongue.

- The 'to feel' aspect of your diagnosis includes pulse diagnosis and feeling your structure. Other aspects are also examined, such as your nails and skin and the temperature on your torso.
- After asking you questions and making observations, your practitioner sifts through this information and pulls it together to create a diagnosis. This forms the basis for your treatment.

9

Common Ailments Seen
the Chinese Way:
Keeping Yourself Healthy

When your acupuncturist asks you about your main complaint
you'll probably give it a name such as 'arthritis', 'high blood
pressure' or 'asthma'. Alternatively you might describe what you
are actually experiencing. For instance, you might complain of
pain or nausea or that you are feeling low and depressed. The
specific questions and observations described in the previous
chapter enable your practitioner to find the cause of your problem.

Chinese medicine recognises that although an illness has the
same name it can arise from many different causes. For example, one person's headache might come from too much Yang Qi
in the Liver and someone else's from the Kidney Qi being deficient. Different people's complaints can have many different
causes.

In this chapter I'll be looking at a number of common conditions and describing how your acupuncturist might diagnose
them. Although I am looking at a number of different named
disorders, please remember that ultimately acupuncture treats

people, not illnesses. In general, one of the first signs that treatment is working is that you'll feel increased well-being and vitality and feel better in yourself.

These are the common illnesses I will deal with in the chapter:

- Anxiety and panic attacks
- Asthma
- Back pain
- Colds and flu
- Constipation
- Depression
- Diarrhoea
- Headaches and migraines
- Hypertension (high blood pressure)
- Indigestion and heartburn
- Insomnia
- Joint pains and musculo-skeletal disorders
- Menopausal hot flushes
- Obesity
- Period pains
- Post-viral syndrome
- Pre-menstrual tension

For each of these conditions, I'll describe how your acupuncturist might diagnose you, how you might be treated, some of the common causes of the problem and some lifestyle advice. I will also include other considerations, such as any special acupuncture techniques or any unusual frequency of visits. These are not, of course, the only conditions that acupuncture can treat (see the end of this chapter for a more detailed list). If you have a condition not mentioned in this book you can ring your local practitioner to find out if it is likely to respond to treatment.

Anxiety and panic attacks

Nearly 16 per cent of the patients seeking treatment at the teaching clinic of the College of Integrated Chinese Medicine come for some kind of psychological problem, including anxiety and panic attacks. You may recall in Chapter 2 that Jenny, a 22-year-old student, was successfully treated for anxiety. Anxiety, fretfulness, panic attacks, apprehension and unease are increasingly common conditions in our angst-ridden society, and acupuncture can be of tremendous benefit.

According to Chinese medicine, anxiety or panic attacks are most often caused by Blood deficiency and Yin deficiency and may affect the Heart and/or the Kidneys.

Chinese medical diagnosis

HEART BLOOD DEFICIENCY

You may remember that your Heart Blood houses your Shen or mind-spirit. If your Blood is deficient, your mind-spirit becomes unsettled, causing anxiety or panic. You may also have other symptoms such as insomnia, palpitations and/or a poor memory and feel extremely vulnerable.

The most common cause of Heart Blood deficiency is stress. If you are already anxious, a vicious circle can form. The Heart Blood deficiency can both cause and be the result of your anxiety. Acupuncture can calm and strengthen you, thus breaking the circle and enabling you to cope with many of the situations that you find so stressful.

You can assist your treatment by putting aside time for relaxation. For example, it is best to ensure that you relax before going to bed and take at least eight hours' rest in bed, even if you have difficulty sleeping. You might also benefit from taking sufficiently long lunch breaks and if possible having a short rest after lunch. By doing this, your body can create better quality Blood. A healthy diet, rich in protein, can also enrich the quality of your Blood.

Your acupuncturist might choose a number of points to benefit your Blood. For example, one point on your mid-back area is a 'special' point for the Blood. Combining this with a point on your Heart or Pericardium channel can settle your Heart and strengthen your Blood, enabling you to feel calmer.

Foods that nourish the Blood

Animal protein, such as red and white meat, poultry and fish, is the most Blood nourishing of all food and unless there is an ethical reason for being vegetarian it is best to eat a small amount every day.

These foods are also helpful for nourishing the Blood:

- **Protein substitutes** – such as tofu and miso.
- **Seaweed products** – some common ones are hiziki, nori and wakame. Seaweed is very nourishing, low in fibre and contains minerals such as potassium, calcium, magnesium and iron as well as iodine.
- **Sprouted beans** – bean sprouts are considered to be energy-enhancing foods.
- **Dried fruits** – such as dates, apricots and figs.
- **Vegetables** – especially leafy, green vegetables.

HEART AND/OR KIDNEY YIN DEFICIENCY

Fear is the emotion associated with the Kidneys. A disturbed Heart will cause you to feel anxious. If the cooling and calming Yin energy is deficient in both your Heart and Kidneys, it is not surprising that you might feel panicky, restless, nervous and/or anxious. Acupuncture treatment, using points to strengthen the Yin energy, can bring these two Organs back to a healthy balance and enable you to relax and settle.

Like Heart Blood deficiency, Heart and Kidney Yin deficiency is most commonly caused by stress. Finding ways to rest and relax will assist your treatment. Relaxing exercises such as Tai Ji Quan, for example, can have a profound effect, enabling you to become calmer and more peaceful. Excessive caffeine from drinking tea, coffee, hot chocolate or cola can also deplete your Heart Yin and can stop you sleeping. If you are drinking excessive amounts of these drinks, your practitioner may suggest that you cut down on your intake.

Asthma

Chinese medicine describes asthma as *xiao*, which means wheezing, combined with *chuan*, which means breathlessness. Each year in the UK, over 18 million working days are lost to asthma and treatment with conventional medicines such as inhalers costs £850 million.[1] Asthma can be very successfully treated with Chinese medicine (see Sarah's case history in Chapter 2) and treatment aims to find the root of the problem rather than palliate the symptoms. This could be much more cost-effective than conventional treatment. Your practitioner is likely to commence with weekly treatments and will suggest that you cut down on any inhalers only if and when you are ready and when your doctor agrees.

Asthma is commonly caused by deficient Lungs or Kidneys, or by Phlegm or Liver Qi stagnation blocking the Lungs. Colds and flu, which Chinese medicine refers to as 'Wind-Cold' or 'Wind-Heat', can exacerbate asthma.

Chinese medical diagnosis

LUNG OR KIDNEY QI DEFICIENCY

Deficient Lung Qi is the most common cause of asthma. You might have symptoms such as feeling weak in your chest, a weak voice and more difficulty breathing out than in. Asthma arising from the Lungs is often worsened by poor posture, especially during childhood. Children (or adults) who stoop over books, sit on wrongly adjusted seats, or watch television or use computers for long periods may not breathe properly because they are putting undue pressure on their chest. Adjusting the posture and encouraging more breaks for activity can help to improve breathing. Grief or sadness can also weaken the Lungs, especially if these feelings are unexpressed over long periods of time. To treat Lung Qi deficiency, your practitioner will strengthen your Lungs with points on your Lung channel and if necessary will use moxibustion to warm the Lungs.

If Kidney deficiency is the cause of asthma, it may be worse when you breathe in. The Kidneys work with the Lungs and 'grasp' the Qi to deepen the breath. If the Kidneys are weak then this deepening is weakened. It is important that anyone with this type of asthma gets enough rest and sleep in order to fully recoup their energy each day. If you have this kind of asthma your acupuncturist will use points that strengthen the Kidneys. Many of the points are located on the legs but will affect your breathing. Because the Lungs and Kidneys work together your acupuncturist may use points from both channels.

PHLEGM

If your asthma is caused by phlegm, the wheezing is usually worse when you lie down. The phlegm accumulates when you are horizontal and you may need propping up with pillows when you sleep. Rather than feeling weak in your chest you may feel full, and may sometimes (although not necessarily) spit up some sticky phlegm. If phlegm is the cause of your asthma, your acupuncturist may advise you to cut down on sticky

Phlegm- and Damp-forming foods, especially dairy produce (see box below). This will assist your acupuncture treatment, which will involve clearing the Phlegm from the Lungs.

LIVER QI STAGNATION

Asthma that becomes worse during emotional upsets or when it is difficult to express feelings like frustration or anger may be due to the Liver. Treatment on your Liver channel can successfully help you to deal with the stress by 'smoothing' and settling your Qi.

WIND-COLD OR WIND-HEAT

Mild asthma can be exacerbated into a full-blown asthma attack by catching a cold or flu. Chinese medical practitioners refer to colds and flu as 'Wind-Cold' or 'Wind-Heat' (see page 193). Acupuncture can clear the Wind-Cold or Wind-Heat, enabling you to recover and bring the asthma back to manageable levels. If it is not cleared, the asthma tends to intensify and this further weakens the already fragile Lungs.

Foods that cause Phlegm and Damp

Some of the most common Damp- and Phlegm-forming foods are:

- Dairy produce – milk, butter, cheese, cream, etc.
- Fatty foods including fatty meat and fried foods
- Sugar and sweeteners
- Wheat – in excess – including bread and pasta
- Concentrated juices such as orange juice, tomato puree
- Excessive alcohol

You might notice that many (but not all) of the foods listed above are 'sticky' in nature. You can start to notice the varying effects different foods have on your system. For many people reducing rather than completely cutting out these foods helps to clear the system. For others – especially if they easily form Phlegm and Damp – it may be best to completely cut these foods from their diet, at least for a while.

Back pain

Chinese medical diagnosis

Backache is one of the commonest complaints seen by an acupuncturist and treatment can be very effective. It is estimated that up to 40 per cent of the British population suffers from back pain in any year[2] and it leads to more time off work than any other problem in the Western world. One reason why acupuncture is so beneficial for this complaint is that Chinese medicine recognises that there are many types of back pain, each with a specific diagnosis. Chinese medicine teaches that the three main reasons for backache are deficient Kidney Qi, Qi and Blood stagnation in the lower back, and Wind, Cold and/or Damp obstructing the lower back.

DEFICIENT KIDNEY QI

If you have a back problem caused by deficient Kidney Qi then you are likely to have a chronic, dull type of backache. The Kidneys are situated in your lower back. If they are functioning sluggishly, a dull ache is created in this area. The ache will often disappear after rest but reappear after further strenuous activity. If you have this kind of backache, your acupuncturist will probably use points that strengthen your Kidneys. For example, a number of points on your lower back can strengthen your Kidney Organs directly. Moxibustion can also be used to warm the area if the deficiency has caused it to become cold.

Emotional problems and over-activity are two important reasons for backache arising from Kidney deficiency. Over-activity carried out under stress causes the muscles to tighten up and any strenuous activity weakens the Kidneys. Getting enough rest, sleeping in a good posture and using chairs that support the spine are all beneficial. Fear is the emotion connected with the Kidneys and chronic fear can lead to weakness in the area of the lower back where they are located. It is worth noting that the Kidneys are associated with the bones and the spine. When people are afraid they often pull away or 'back off' from things. Over time this can affect their posture and weaken the back.

QI AND BLOOD 'STAGNATION' IN THE LOWER BACK

This kind of back problem is severe and painful, but fortunately short-lived – it lasts for only days, or weeks at the most. If it is not treated, however, it can be the precursor of more long-term, chronic back problems. Fortunately, it responds exceptionally well to acupuncture.

The initial cause of this condition is often mental or physical overstrain. People develop tense muscles in the lower back as they try to cope with their problems or strain themselves physically. This prevents their Qi and Blood from moving, which leads to the pain. The pain can develop slowly or the back can suddenly become 'sprained' and a person is unable to move. Anyone who has suffered from this acute sprain will testify to its extreme pain.

Your practitioner will usually use a number of different points to treat this condition – most are not on the back at all. For example, one useful point that can clear this condition lies at the back of the knee. I have often seen this point immediately free up a back pain. Another two points are called 'lower back pain' and lie on the hand. Often you will need a course of four to five treatments, but one treatment will start off the healing process.

WIND, COLD AND/OR DAMP IN THE LOWER BACK

This can cause acute or chronic back pain and is due to these pathogens entering the back directly. For example, when you are gardening you may build up a sweat and remove some of your clothes. As you cool down afterwards, the Wind, Cold and Damp can enter the back through the open pores. Cold causes the tissues to contract, creating pain, and the Wind and Damp also contribute. Similar conditions affect people working on building sites, sunning themselves on a hot day that turns cool, or after exercising and working up a sweat.

To remove the obstructing pathogen, your practitioner can use points in the area, or use cupping (see page 230) to draw the blood to the surface and draw out the pathogen.

A Wind, Cold, Damp backache

My patient, Frances, limped stiffly into the treatment room holding her back. She had woken up with a severe backache and had come for an emergency treatment. She was brought in by her boyfriend. They'd been away for the weekend and had gone rowing on the canal. Afterwards they lay down exhausted on the grass. 'It was lovely sunshine and I really enjoyed it. I'm used to exercising – so I can't understand why it's happened.'

I asked Frances a few more questions and confirmed to myself that the problem was not related to the amount of exercise she'd done. Frances had grown hot when rowing and her pores had opened as she sweated. When she had then lain down on the grass, the Cold and Damp had entered her back through the pores. Frances admitted that the grass had been slightly damp.

I used cupping therapy on her back to treat her. (For more on cupping see Chapter 10.) This drew out the Wind, Cold and Damp. I also used some Bladder channel points on her feet. The Bladder channel runs up the back and the points loosened it. I was certain that my diagnosis was accurate, but was still delighted with the result. It was a miracle – her back pain went immediately! She too was delighted. A check-up and another treatment two days later ensured that the treatment held.

PHYSICAL TRAUMA

A sports injury or an accident is a common cause of back problems and this can also be treated very effectively by acupuncture.

Colds and flu

When you are healthy you have strong 'Wei' Qi or defensive Qi. This defensive Qi lies just between the skin and muscles and protects you from the invasion of Wind from the environment. Colds and flu are either caused by Wind–Cold or Wind–Heat.

Chinese medical diagnosis

WIND-COLD

This gives you symptoms such as a runny nose with clear white mucus, an itchy throat, sneezing, coughing, a slight headache at the base of the skull, a desire to keep warm and/or slightly aching joints.

WIND-HEAT

This is often more severe and similar to flu. You might feel hot and feverish as well as sweaty and thirsty and have swollen tonsils or a sore throat. You might also have a stuffy or runny nose with yellow mucus, fairly severe joint pains and a desire to keep warm. For more about Wind–Cold and Heat and how to protect yourself from these pathogens see Chapter 5.

If you start to become ill with a cold it is best to drop everything and rest. This will often stop the cold from developing. If the cold does develop it is advisable to take time off work to convalesce. By recovering your health before returning to work, you are less vulnerable to repeated infections. It also saves your work colleagues from becoming infected and prevents an epidemic from spreading all around the building.

Treatment

People rarely come for treatment with colds or flu as a main complaint. If you are already having treatment and come in with an infection, however, your acupuncturist will usually use some points to clear it. If you have treatment at the early stages of the infection, it can be very effective. If you have had the infection for a few days, then acupuncture may be less effective.

Your acupuncturist will deal with Wind-Cold or Wind-Heat by using points that are mostly on your upper body. These will be chosen for their specific effect. For example, one point close to the wrist will directly clear the throat, another on the hand will clear symptoms from the face and nose and another at the back of the neck will clear Wind from the neck and eyes. If you have a head cold that is giving you a sore throat, aching eyes and a runny nose these might be a perfect combination. If you have Wind-Cold your acupuncturist might also use cups on your back. These will open the pores, helping you to sweat and thus release the infection.

Constipation

It is normal to open our bowels regularly every day. If you open them less frequently or have difficulty expelling the stool then you are constipated. Some people can only open their bowels with the help of laxatives. If this is the case it is better to find natural ways to open them and become less dependent on pills.

Constipation has many causes. Your practitioner might diagnose the problem as due to deficiency, fullness or obstruction.

Chinese medical diagnosis

'DEFICIENT' CONDITIONS

Two main causes of constipation arise from deficient conditions. They are Spleen Qi deficiency and Blood deficiency. If your Spleen Qi is deficient this can cause your bowel to become sluggish so that the food is not moved or transformed. Blood deficiency usually arises because the Blood is not moistening your system.

If you have a deficient condition causing constipation your acupuncturist will use strengthening acupuncture treatments to help you. She or he may also use moxibustion to warm the lower abdomen. At the same time as treating you, your acupuncturist might also suggest changes to your diet. For example, it is best if your diet is well balanced and full of fresh vegetables, whole grains, beans and fruit. This diet will provide fibre that is essential to normal bowel movements. Those who have a tendency to constipation need to beware of eating processed food or 'fast food', which contain very little fibre and nourishment.

'FULL' CONDITIONS

If the Liver or the Large Intestine are not functioning well, your Qi may stagnate, causing constipation. This may be due to harbouring emotions or 'holding on' to feelings, especially anger, resentment or frustration – but also grief, sadness or other emotions. A static lifestyle can cause this kind of constipation too. Regular light exercise is important for anyone who is constipated, as it encourages bowel movements.

Constipation can also be due to Heat or Cold in the Large Intestine. Heat in the lower abdomen dries up the stool, causing constipation. Cold in the Intestine causes movement to slow down and the bowels to become less active. Alongside acupuncture, diet can help these kinds of constipation. For example, some foods such as red meats, curries and spices should be avoided if there is Heat. Cooling foods such as cold salads, many fruits, iced drinks and any food that comes straight from the fridge should not be eaten if there is Cold. (See the box below for more on temperatures of food.)

Acupuncture treatment can be used to clear any of the above 'full' conditions. It can move the obstruction so that the bowels can work properly again. If Cold has caused the bowel problem then your practitioner will usually warm the lower abdomen with a moxa stick or moxa box.

Hot, warm, neutral, cool and cold foods[3]

Hot	Black pepper, butter, chicken fat, chocolate, coffee, crispy rice, curry, hot chillies, lamb, onions, sesame seeds, smoked fish, trout, whisky and other spirits.
Warm	Beef, black-eyed beans, brown sugar, cheese, chestnuts, chicken meat, dates, egg yolk, garlic, ginger, green (bell) peppers, ham, leeks, lobster, mussels, oats, peaches, peanut butter, peanuts, pomegranates, potatoes, prawns, shrimps, turkey, vinegar, walnuts, wine.
Neutral	Aduki beans, apricots, beetroot, black tea, bread, broad beans, brown rice, cabbage, carrots, cherries, corn, egg white, chickpeas (garbanzos), dates, grapes, honey, hot water, lentils, kidney beans, milk, oysters, peas, plums, pork, raisins, red beans, rye, salmon, sugar, sweet potatoes, turnips.
Cool	Almonds, apples, asparagus, barley, broccoli, cabbage, cauliflower, celery, chicory, corn, fish, mushrooms, mangoes, mung beans, oranges, pears, pineapple, radishes,

rhubarb, salt, seaweed, soya beans, spinach, strawberries, tangerines, wheat, wild rice.

Cold   Bananas, bean sprouts, cucumber, duck, grapefruit, green tea, lettuce, ice cream, peppermint, sorbet, tofu, tomatoes, water melon, yoghurt.

Depression

Depression can vary from low-grade gloom and sadness to a condition so debilitating that it is impossible to move or function without help. It can initially be brought on by outside circumstances such as a relationship break-up, the death of a loved one, difficulties at work or financial worries, but sometimes the cause is not clear. Once in this state it is often difficult for a person to recover without outside help. Chinese medicine teaches that there are many causes of depression. Below are the most common 'full' and 'deficient' causes.

Chinese medical diagnosis

'FULL' CONDITIONS

There are two main 'full' conditions that cause depression: stagnation of the Liver Qi and Dampness. By far the most common cause of depression is stagnation of the Liver Qi. The Liver is responsible for keeping your Qi flowing smoothly throughout your system. If you become frustrated, angry, resentful or hold in your emotions this may cause the emotions to implode and your Qi to stop flowing freely, thus causing depression. If the implosion is recognised and your feelings articulated, it will often help to clear it. As well as giving you treatment, your acupuncturist will usually support you and encourage you to talk about your problems and worries.

Depression caused by stagnation of the Liver Qi will often lift if you get moving. Any exercise is helpful, including brisk walking, swimming, playing a racket game or Tai Ji Quan. Someone who is feeling low does not always find it easy to get up and start exercising. Once they start moving, however, and the energy starts flowing again, they usually feel better.

When your acupuncturist treats you, she or he will use points to clear obstruction from the Liver channel. Some of these points move the Qi, while others lift the spirits. For example, one very effective point that lies on the torso is called 'the Gate of Hope'. This point can have a profound effect on a person's mind-spirit and enable her or him to find renewed hope for the future.

Dampness is another cause of depression. It can clog up the system and obstruct the Qi. Some people with Dampness are also affected by damp weather and find that they become more depressed when the weather is gloomy for long periods. People who live in damp houses can also become depressed. A dehumidifier in the house helps to clear the dampness from the environment. This may in turn brighten the spirits. Your practitioner will often use points on your Stomach and Spleen channels to clear Dampness.

'EMPTY' CONDITIONS

There are many 'empty' conditions that can cause depression. The most common ones are Heart, Pericardium or Lung Qi deficiency. If your Heart or Pericardium Qi is weak you may feel dull and lacking in joy and vitality. If your Lung Qi is weak you may become depleted and depressed because you are unable to revitalise your Lungs with fresh air. The depression can come about if you have a severe emotional upset, such as a relationship break-up or bereavement, that exacerbates an existing Heart or Lung weakness.

Your acupuncturist will treat you by strengthening points along your Heart, Pericardium and/or Lung channels. If necessary, she or he will also use points that support your mind-spirit. For example, a point on your arm called 'the Heavenly Spring' will strengthen, calm and lighten your mind-spirit and help you to feel more relaxed and open in your chest area.

Diarrhoea

It is normal to pass a well-formed stool every day. If the stools are semi-formed or watery and you open your bowels more than once or twice a day then you have diarrhoea. If you have chronic diarrhoea you will not get enough nourishment from your food and over a long period of time this weakens your Qi. Chinese medicine finds many causes for diarrhoea. Some of the most common ones are associated with your Spleen, because it rules your digestion and transforms your food and fluids.

Chinese medical diagnosis

DEFICIENT SPLEEN QI

If your Spleen is weak it can no longer transform and move your food, so your food passes straight through your intestines.

One cause of Spleen Qi deficiency is eating too much cold food. The Chinese say that the Spleen likes 'warmth'. Too much cold food, such as iced drinks, salads, yoghurt or fruit, stops the Spleen from working efficiently and your food is then not digested well. It is better to take food or drink at room temperature. Excessive amounts of sweet sugary food also weaken the Spleen and this can exacerbate loose bowels. It is best to avoid fast food or other poor-quality food as these weaken the Spleen too. Overwork, Dampness or excessive worrying can also cause Spleen Qi deficiency.

Acupuncture treatment on the Spleen can have a strongly beneficial effect on your bowels. Your practitioner might use acupuncture points located on your legs and feet as well as points on your abdomen. She or he might also use moxibustion to warm the Spleen.

DAMPNESS

Dampness can be compared to muddy water stuck inside us. It can block the Spleen's ability to move and transform your food and drink. Sometimes the Damp combines with Cold in the body, causing a watery stool and some abdominal pain. Damp can also combine with Heat and the stool then has a strong odour and is watery and yellow.

Climatic conditions that are hot and damp can often cause this Damp-Heat type of loose bowels. These often occur, for example, when people take holidays in hot, damp countries. Acute and extremely foul-smelling diarrhoea can also be caused by greasy and heating food. This may include strong curries or excessive fatty meat such as lamb or beef. It can also be caused by eating unclean food.

If diarrhoea has been caused by these pathogens then your acupuncturist will need to clear the obstruction. If you have an acute condition of Dampness you may need a few treatments every other day in order to fully clear the condition. A more chronic condition will require less frequent treatments, often at weekly intervals but over a longer period of time.

STAGNANT LIVER QI COMBINED WITH A WEAK SPLEEN

If you have this condition you may have alternating constipation and diarrhoea. It is often caused and made worse by worry, nervousness, anger and anxiety. If you are worried or slightly stressed for a short time, for example, this can cause an episode of loose bowels. This clears once the stress is cleared. If you are under constant stress in your home or work situation this can result in chronic diarrhoea that can be very depleting. To treat the condition your acupuncturist will smooth and settle the Liver Qi as well as strengthening your Spleen Qi. Treating the two Organs together can calm you so that in turn your bowels also settle.

Headaches and migraines

Headaches and migraines are very common complaints. It is estimated that in the United States up to 50 million people go to the doctor complaining of headaches per year.[4] Happily, acupuncture can be very beneficial for this condition. Headaches come in many forms. They can occur on different areas of the head, with varying types of pain and be experienced at a range of intensities. The two most common triggers for headaches are diet and stress, although general lifestyle can also be important. One simple way of classifying headaches is to notice whether they are 'full' in their nature or 'empty'.

Chinese medical diagnosis

A 'FULL' HEADACHE

People often describe the pain from these headaches as throbbing, stabbing, pulling, distending or heavy. The pains are often severe and if the headache is very debilitating it might be called a migraine. Chinese medicine teaches that such headaches often arise from over-activity of the Liver but they can also be caused by Dampness.

Headaches caused by the Liver are varied and can be situated on the temples, at the sides or top of the head or behind the eyes. These kinds of headaches are often a 'message' that you are under stress. If frustration and anger, excessive worrying, anxiety or fear go unexpressed over a period of time they can build up until they explode into a headache. Some women get headaches before a period, when they are most tense. Other people find that they get headaches after the source of stress is over and when they are resting, so often this is at the weekend or on holidays. Coffee, tea and alcohol can also set off headaches – anyone who suffers from headaches and drinks alcohol and caffeinated drinks should try cutting them from their diet. Some headaches are exacerbated by food allergies.

A headache originating from Dampness can create a heavy feeling on the forehead. A diet full of Damp-forming foods such as dairy produce or rich and greasy food can be the cause of this kind of headache. (See page 189 for a list of these foods.)

Acupuncture can often successfully treat these kinds of headaches and migraines. If the headache is due to a full Liver, for example, your practitioner might use a point situated at the base of the neck that will directly affect your eyes and head. This may be coupled with points on the Liver and Gall Bladder channels of your feet. Together these clear your Liver and help to move the obstructed Qi. Because there are so many causes for migraines, your practitioner will often work with you to isolate anything that is exacerbating the headaches and, where appropriate, she or he will suggest lifestyle changes.

Patrick's migraine treatment

Patrick was a patient of one of my colleagues. He came to be treated for migraines. He was 56 years old and managed a laundry. His job was very stressful. Before having acupuncture he had had so many different treatments that he didn't have any belief in a cure. 'I decided to try acupuncture as there weren't any other treatments left! I've tried homeopathy, reflexology, aromatherapy and osteopathy. I'd also taken many painkillers.' He no longer needs to take painkillers now.

He described the pain as severe and throbbing. It was on the right-hand side of his head and travelled over to his right eye. The pain would last for anything from two or three days to a week. The migraines varied in severity and were either 'uncomfortable', 'very uncomfortable' or 'evil'. The evil ones appeared once every three months.

His practitioner diagnosed that the headaches came from fullness in his Liver. At the first treatment she placed needles into four points in his feet and left them in place for about 20 minutes. There was such a vast improvement in his headaches that after four or five visits he stopped treatment. His practitioner had warned him that he wasn't completely better, however, and after one month his headaches returned. 'I put up with it for a while then I had one that lasted for five weeks. It was terrible. I finally went back for more treatment and my headache went the next day!'

Patrick has been having treatment for a year now and goes once a month. 'I occasionally have a mild migraine but only about once every few months. My circumstances are no different and my job is still as pressurised as before but now I'm much more relaxed – other people have commented on it as well.'

A 'DEFICIENT' HEADACHE

This is often described as a weak, dull or 'empty' headache. 'Deficient' headaches are often due to deficient Qi, especially in the Kidneys, or they can be due to Blood deficiency. The pain is less intense than 'full' headaches but can last longer. They often manifest as an empty feeling inside the head, at the back of the neck, on the forehead or at the top of the head. Overworking can weaken your Qi and/or Blood and cause these headaches. Diet can also play a part in causing such headaches and it may be important to eat a diet rich in Blood-nourishing foods, especially meat, poultry and fish.

When treating this kind of headache your acupuncturist will strengthen the Qi of your Kidneys or any other imbalanced Organ or may nourish your Blood by treating appropriate points on your Spleen or Liver.

Hypertension (high blood pressure)

Headaches, dizziness, irritability and a slight ringing in the ears are all signals that your blood pressure might be high. More often people don't have any obvious signs and symptoms. They often discover that their blood pressure is high when they have it measured by their doctor or other health practitioner. It has been estimated that approximately 20 per cent of the UK population has high blood pressure.[5] If left unchecked, chronic high blood pressure can in the long term cause a stroke or a heart attack, so it is essential for people to have it monitored and treated. Acupuncture is one therapy that can be very helpful in its treatment and Chinese medicine identifies a number of different causes. Three major ones are over-activity of Yang energy, Phlegm, and Deficient Kidney Qi. These syndromes may be found separately or together. The most common lifestyle causes of hypertension are a combination of stress, diet and a lack of rest and relaxation.

Chinese medical diagnosis

OVER-ACTIVITY OF THE 'YANG' ENERGY

Yang energy moves and warms you, while Yin energy cools and settles you down. Stress, which causes a person to become frustrated, resentful or explosively angry, can be a major reason for hypertension and may cause the Yang energy to become over-active and raise the blood pressure. Overworking can also be a cause, by putting the body under strain. In this case hypertension is a signal that you should reassess the way that you are working and relax more. When treating you for hypertension your acupuncturist will use points to clear excess Heat and settle the Liver. Over time this can bring your blood pressure down.

PHLEGM

Phlegm can fur up the arteries and is similar to arteriosclerosis in Western medicine. Cutting out Phlegm- and Damp-forming foods, especially dairy produce such as milk, butter and cheese, as well as fatty meat products and any other rich food such as mayonnaise, ice cream, and rich cakes and biscuits, can help to lower the blood pressure. Your acupuncturist can use points to clear the Phlegm directly as well as strengthen the Spleen.

DEFICIENT KIDNEY QI

Weakened Kidney Qi can also cause hypertension. Salt is the taste associated with the Kidneys and cutting down can often be beneficial. Salt regulates the water balance in the body but in large quantities it will stress the Heart and Kidneys and intensify high blood pressure. Acupuncture treatment will be carried out to strengthen the Kidneys directly.

Indigestion and heartburn

Symptoms of indigestion include discomfort and/or pain in the stomach or chest area, feeling full, sour regurgitation and belching. If you've ever eaten late then woken in the middle of the night with excruciating stomach pain, you've experienced acute indigestion. If it is more chronic it often comes on after a heavy meal. Indigestion is most commonly due to food stagnating in the Stomach, or the Liver Qi becoming stagnant. In both of these cases the normal digestive process has temporarily stopped.

Chinese medical diagnosis

FOOD STAGNATING IN THE STOMACH OR LIVER QI STAGNATION

Some people with digestive problems find themselves in situations that they find hard to sort out and 'digest'. For example, unexpressed anger and resentment can cause your digestion to slow down or come to a standstill. If you are gripped by anxiety, fear, worry or dread this can affect the solar plexus and stomach. This may also cause the digestive process to come to a temporary standstill.

Anyone who frequently gets indigestion is advised to examine their diet. If the diet contains a high percentage of rich food then reducing this can help to alleviate the problem. Indigestion can also be caused by over-eating, in which case the diet needs to be modified. Those who get indigestion should strive to eat in situations which are as stress free and as calm as possible and to continue to relax for a little while after eating in order to aid the digestive process.

Your acupuncturist will treat this problem by using points to clear obstructions in your Liver and Stomach channels. Ren 12, which lies in the centre of your Stomach, is an acupuncture point you may instinctively massage when you have this problem. Your practitioner will probably strengthen any underlying weakness in your Stomach's 'rotting and ripening' function so that you can more easily digest your food.

Insomnia

Insomnia is the inability to get off to sleep, or waking in the night having initially fallen asleep.

The most common causes of insomnia are due to the Heart being unsettled, and Heat.

Chinese medicine diagnosis

HEART YIN OR BLOOD DEFICIENCY

If the Yin energy or the Blood of your Heart is deficient it will cause the Shen to become unsettled, in turn causing insomnia. If you have Heart Blood deficiency you are likely to have difficulty getting off to sleep. Heart Yin deficiency causes a person to wake up for periods in the middle of the night – often having previously dropped off to sleep without any difficulty.

If you have insomnia caused by Heart Yin or Blood deficiency it may be exacerbated by dietary factors, overworking and/or being generally over-stimulated. For example, eating irregularly, over-eating or eating late at night can cause you to wake because your stomach is trying to digest food when it should be resting. People who overwork, especially in a stressful environment, often find that when they go to bed they can't sleep. Before going to bed it is important to relax. Strenuous exercise, watching a scary film or reading over-stimulating books can prevent a person from winding down. Drinking coffee, tea, cola or other caffeinated drinks can also prevent people from sleeping.

If insomnia is due to Heart Yin or Blood deficiency you may also have other symptoms such as anxiety, palpitations and a poor memory. If this is the cause, some of the points your practitioner will treat will be on the Heart channel on your arms and hands, in order to settle your Shen.

HEAT

If you've ever lain awake on a hot summer night you know how heat can keep you from sleeping. Internal Heat can have a number of different causes including Heat in the Liver, the Stomach or the Heart. Too much hot food such as curry, red meat or alcohol can make this worse. Your practitioner will use points to clear the Heat as well as other points to treat the underlying cause. At the same time as clearing the Heat she or he may also treat your Yin energy.

Joint pains and musculo-skeletal disorders

When I was in China I was impressed to see that the local acupuncturist was often the first port of call for many patients with joint pains. Treatment for these conditions can be very successful. Over 25 per cent of patients who have treatment at the student clinic of the College of Integrated Chinese Medicine come with these kinds of problems. The term 'joint pains and musculo-skeletal disorders' covers a large number of conditions including rheumatoid arthritis, osteo-arthritis, bursitis, fibrositis, injured joints, etc.

Chinese medicine views musculo-skeletal conditions differently from Western medicine. It categorises them according to the type of pain. This pain may be due to either a 'full' or 'deficient' condition. Many joint pains are caused by pathogens such as Wind, Cold, Damp, Heat and also Phlegm. In this case they are 'full' in nature and the pain may be strong. If they are caused by Blood or Qi deficiency then the joint pains are duller and ache more.

Chinese medical diagnosis

'FULL' JOINT PAINS

Wind in the joints is characterised by pain in the muscles and joints that moves from place to place, while Cold causes severe pain in the joints that causes limitation of movement. Dampness in the joints is characterised by stiffness and swelling, along with a feeling of heaviness in the joint or limb. Heat in the joints causes them to become red, swollen, hot and painful.

Phlegm nodules form in joints when the fluids dry up. This usually occurs in joints that have been affected for a long period of time. Qi and Blood stagnation in the joints is often caused by trauma and is characterised by quite severe pain.

If your joint problems are caused by Wind, Damp, Cold and/or Heat you are likely to be susceptible to the correspond-ing climate. For example, if you have Damp in your joints you might dislike damp or humid weather and may even know when the weather is turning damp because of the aching sensa-tion you experience. Windy or cold weather can exacerbate joint pains in the same way. Extremely hot weather can worsen red, hot, swollen joints.

When your acupuncturist treats your joint pains she or he will often choose points that are close to the site of your pain as well as ones that are further from it. The points close to the pain will directly clear any local blockages of Wind, Cold and Damp in the channels. Other distal points are used to strengthen any underlying deficiency.

'DEFICIENT' JOINT PAINS

Joint pains due to Qi and Blood deficiency can affect many different Organs, especially your Liver, Kidneys and Spleen. Deficiency causes the joints to ache rather than become painful. The limbs may also feel weak. If the ache is a general one it may be because there is a generalised Qi or Blood deficiency throughout the body. This may have various causes, including overwork, poor diet or emotional difficulties. Sometimes joint problems are caused by overuse of one particular area. For example, someone who is constantly carrying heavy loads may be affected in the hips, or someone working on a computer may find repetitive strain injury (RSI) affecting the hands and wrists.

If you have joint pains due to deficiency your acupuncturist may advise you to get plenty of rest and to eat well. She or he will stimulate and strengthen the weakened Organs and channels. Many people with joint pains have a mixture of a 'deficient' and 'full' condition and in such a case your practitioner will both clear the obstruction and strengthen the Organs that are Qi and/or Blood deficient.

Doreen's obstructed shoulder

Doreen told me that she was usually tough. She had worked in the mills for 40 years and had learned that if a problem came along you either do something about it or forget it. She decided to try acupuncture with one of my colleagues. 'I'd had a frozen shoulder for six months. It appeared within a day and a half and I still don't know where it came from. I was restricted in every way and I couldn't bear to spend the rest of my life in pain. I couldn't comb my hair, pull out a drawer or grip anything – the pain just shot from my shoulder to my thumb. I was so desperate that life wasn't worth living. I'd got very down and depressed, it was shocking.'

Doreen's acupuncturist diagnosed that her problem lay in the energy connected to her Large Intestine channel. This channel runs along the outside of the arm and over the shoulder and it had become blocked. Treatment was aimed at removing the blockage.

Doreen's underlying Qi needed strengthening and her practitioner found that she had a weakness in the Qi of her chest that affected mainly her Lungs but also her Heart Qi. The Lungs and Large Intestine are connected and the underlying deficiency in her Lung energy had probably caused stagnation in her Large Intestine channel, so it was important both to remove the blockage and to strengthen her energy.

'I went in January and even after the first treatment it eased. After three times the difference was amazing and since then it's got better and better! Now I can use my arm for anything and I've even painted and decorated the kitchen. I do get a very slight ache still if I use an area behind my shoulder but I don't normally feel it. I've really gone back to being how I was. I'd also had a bad back from a fall and that got better too – I've never had the pain since. Now I say, don't be put off by acupuncture, you don't know until you've tried it. Whatever it cost me it's been worth every penny.'

Menopausal hot flushes

Kidney Yin deficiency is the most common cause of menopausal hot flushes although the Liver and/or the Heart may also be involved.

Chinese medicine diagnosis

KIDNEY YIN DEFICIENCY

Yin is cooling, moistening and calming. Yang on the other hand is heating, drying and moving. As people grow older they need to rest appropriately. Many people continue to overwork when they need to rest and this uses up their Yin energy. They are left with too little of this cooling energy and too much hot energy, causing hot flushes. It is now normal for many people to over-work in ways they never did before, and when hot flushes first appear it can be a signal that you need to rest. It is interesting to note that hot flushes are less common in China, where people generally have less stressful working lives, than they are in the

West. As China takes on the habits of Western society this is likely to change. Diet, a hot climate and emotional stress can all intensify hot flushes.

Acupuncture can be very helpful in the treatment of hot flushes and your practitioner will usually clear the Heat as well as nourishing and strengthening your Kidneys. Treatment is not always effective straight away but it can work extremely quickly.

Obesity

Nearly two-thirds of adults in the United States are over-weight and over 30 per cent are classified as obese.[6] The UK is catching up fast with over half the population either over-weight or obese. Obesity in children between two and four years old almost doubled between 1989 and 1998 and in a similar period it trebled in 6 to 15-year-olds. If current trends continue, conservative estimates are that at least one-third of adults, one-fifth of boys and one-third of girls will be obese by 2020.[7] Many people hope that acupuncture can give them a 'quick fix' cure. Although acupuncture can help people who are overweight, most acupuncturists will only carry out treat-ment that deals with the underlying cause of the problem. Treatment that suppresses the appetite is not useful. Unless the cause is dealt with, a person will go back to old habits and the weight will pile back on as soon as the treatment is stopped.

Chinese medicine correlates overweight with Dampness col-lecting in the body. This may be due to an underlying defi-ciency in the Spleen or Kidneys although it can also arise from an imbalance in other Organs.

Chinese medical diagnosis

DAMPNESS AND SPLEEN OR KIDNEY DEFICIENCY

Damp arises when the Spleen, Stomach and/or Kidneys fail to transform the Body Fluids. If the Spleen and Stomach are weak they may turn your food and fluid into fat instead of allowing them to nourish you. Over-eating or a poor diet can also weaken the Spleen and Stomach. A vicious circle of poor eating habits leading to a weak Spleen and Stomach, coupled with their inability to transform your food, can create many weight problems. If the Kidneys are at the root of a weight problem they can cause the body to hold water and thus add weight.

IMBALANCE IN OTHER ORGANS

Many other imbalances can lie behind a weight problem. For instance, if the weight problem is due to over-eating this can have many causes. People who have a Heart or Pericardium problem may feel unloved, for example, and may 'comfort eat' to make themselves feel better. People with Lung imbalances may over-eat to fill a sense of emptiness inside. By treating the cause of these problems the weight problem can also be dealt with. People will then not only return to a more normal weight but will also feel better in themselves.

If you have treatment for a weight problem your acupuncturist will usually also discuss your eating habits and diet and, if necessary, make other lifestyle suggestions that will assist the treatment.

Some suggestions to support your healthy weight loss
- **Eat nourishing food but avoid dieting.** The correct dietary proportions vary slightly for each individual but in general a nourishing diet contains approximately
  40–45% grains and beans
  40–45% fresh vegetables and fruit

15–20% 'rich' foods such as meat, poultry, eggs, dairy, fats (eg olive oil, coconut oil or flax oil) and sugars.

Some people prefer to take slightly less grains and beans and more fruit and vegetables. It is best to eat organic food if possible and avoid foods that contain additives. A healthy diet will strengthen the Spleen and allow it to work at maximum capacity.

- **Eat three meals a day regularly.** Skipping meals weakens the Spleen. If you skip breakfast your energy levels may drop later in the morning. This can cause cravings for chocolate or other sugary snacks.
- **Cut down on Damp- and Phlegm-forming food.** These rich foods are sticky and difficult to digest and put a strain on the Spleen and Stomach. (See box on page 189 listing Phlegm- and Damp-forming foods.) Many people find that they effortlessly lose weight when they cut down or cut out wheat.
- **Avoid cold foods and drink.** This can be a major cause of weight problems. Cold slows movement down, while heat speeds it up. Taking foodstuffs such as iced drinks, frozen yoghurts or too many raw vegetables slows the metabolism.
- **Avoid eating too much overly sweet food.** The sweet taste is associated with the Spleen. A moderate amount of the sweet taste is very strengthening but an excess weakens the Spleen. It is best to cut down on extremely sweet-tasting food and to avoid food sweetened with sugar altogether.
- **Start doing moderate exercise.** When we cut down on food the body thinks there is a famine and starts to conserve our food and energy. To lose weight we need to exercise, which speeds up the metabolism.

Period pains

Chinese medicine describes many different types of period pains. The main ones are due to Cold in the lower abdomen, stagnation of Qi in the lower abdomen and stagnation of Blood in the lower abdomen. When treating this condition your practitioner will ensure you have at least three pain-free periods before she or he is satisfied that your pain has completely cleared.

Chinese medical diagnosis

COLD IN THE LOWER ABDOMEN

Pains from Cold are sharp and 'biting' in nature. They often feel better with the application of heat. These pains can often be caused by leaving the lower abdomen uncovered so that the cold 'invades'. Alternatively they may be due to walking around without shoes. The cold then enters the channels of the legs and travels up to the lower abdomen. If you have this kind of period pain it is essential to protect yourself from Cold. It may also be important to avoid sex during your period because the uterus is at its most fragile at this time and is more susceptible to Cold.

This type of period pain will often respond to a combination of moxibustion and needles. Your practitioner may use a moxa stick on the lower abdomen. Both acute and chronic period pains can be helped. Acute pains can be greatly eased by placing a warming moxa box on your lower abdomen.

STAGNATION OF QI IN THE LOWER ABDOMEN

Period pains characterised by a distended (bloated) feeling are often due to stagnation of the Qi in the lower abdomen. Rubbing the stuck area encourages the Qi to move, helping to alleviate the pain. This kind of period pain is often exacerbated if a person is living or working in a stressful situation. Your practitioner will often use a combination of points to move the Qi in the lower abdomen and may want to give you treatments a few days before your period is due.

STAGNATION OF BLOOD IN THE LOWER ABDOMEN

Some period pains are extremely intense and do not easily respond to massage or heat. These may be accompanied by blood clots. They are often due to Blood that is stuck in the lower abdomen. This kind of period pain is the most difficult of the three types to treat and your acupuncturist will use special points aimed at moving your Blood in your lower abdomen.

Post-viral syndrome

Post-viral syndrome or myalgic encephalomyelitis (commonly known as ME) is now a frequent cause of chronic illness. A person with this syndrome (see Samantha's case history in Chapter 2) can experience a wide variety of symptoms including muscle fatigue and aches, poor memory and concentration, exhaustion and an intermittent but persistent flu-like feeling. This condition is usually caused by Wind, Cold, Heat or Damp combined with Qi and Blood deficiency.

Chinese medical diagnosis

WIND, COLD, HEAT OR DAMP PLUS QI AND BLOOD DEFICIENCY

People who get this condition are often chronically overworking and weakening their body's energy. If they then become ill from an infection or virus (an invasion of Wind, Cold, Heat or Damp in Chinese medicine), they may not be strong enough to throw it off because their underlying Qi and Blood is weak. Proper rest during the illness and then taking time to convalesce gives the body the chance to regain its strength so that it can throw off the pathogen/virus. A healthy diet is also important. This condition often occurs in people who are overachievers or who overwork and these people may find it difficult to cut down on their activities.

Acupuncture treatment can be extremely helpful for people with this condition. Your acupuncturist will use points to clear the underlying pathogen and at the same time to strengthen your Qi and Blood. Some people recover from the condition more rapidly than others and the path to health can be somewhat uneven – many people take two steps forward and one back. Patients should record their overall progress over a period of weeks and months to keep them motivated if they go through any temporary setbacks.

Pre-menstrual syndrome

The main symptoms of this condition are fluctuating moods, depression or anger before the period, tender or swollen breasts and a swollen abdomen. Women usually begin to feel pre-menstrual three to four days before their period begins. Sometimes pre-menstrual tension can start as early as two weeks before a period. In this case it is very debilitating. The main cause of pre-menstrual syndrome is stagnation of the Liver Qi, although deficiency of the Blood or Yin can also be involved.

Chinese medical diagnosis

STAGNATION OF LIVER QI

The Liver is responsible for the smooth and even movement of Qi throughout the body. If the Liver is not smoothing the Qi it moves unevenly, causing people to feel erratic, angry and irritable, as well as having the symptoms described above.

Those who have pre-menstrual syndrome may notice that the intensity of the symptoms varies according to the intensity of the stress in the week preceding the period. They might also notice that light exercise improves the symptoms, as does resting for half an hour every day. Rest can help to relax a person and allow the Liver Qi to move. Cutting out caffeinated drinks can help to lessen the effects of pre-menstrual syndrome.

Many people who have had acupuncture will attest to its effectiveness in treating pre-menstrual tension. Your acupuncturist may clear the stagnation a few days before the tension begins and then support any underlying Qi deficiency just after the period finishes.

Some other conditions acupuncture is often used to treat

Acupuncture can help many conditions in addition to the above complaints. Below are the other general complaints for which patients most commonly come for treatment:

- **Breathing and lung problems** such as chronic breathlessness, bronchitis, coughs, hayfever.
- **Circulatory problems** such as angina, chronic heart conditions, low blood pressure, palpitations, poor circulation, stroke, thrombosis, varicose veins.
- **Digestive and bowel complaints** such as inflamed gall bladder, gall stones, gastritis, nausea, stomach ulcers, vomiting, colitis, dysentery, irritable bowel syndrome.
- **Ear, eye, nose, mouth and throat disorders** such as blurred vision, chronic catarrh, conjunctivitis, deafness, dry eyes, gum problems, nosebleeds, otitis media, sinusitis, sore throats, tinnitus, tonsillitis, tooth problems.
- **Emotional and mental conditions** such as anxiety, depression, eating disorders, insomnia, panic attacks.
- **Gynaecological disorders** such as heavy periods, irregular, scanty or absent periods, morning sickness, post-natal depression, vaginal discharge.
- **Joint problems and pain** such as osteo-arthritis, rheumatoid arthritis, rheumatism, sciatica, Still's disease.

- **Neurological problems** such as Bell's palsy, epilepsy, multiple sclerosis, neuralgia.
- **Skin conditions** such as acne, eczema, psoriasis, urticaria.
- **Sudden acute disorders** such as food poisoning, stomach upsets, mumps.
- **Urinary and reproductive problems** such as bedwetting, cystitis, impotence, urine retention, incontinence, infertility, kidney stones, prostate conditions.

Conclusion

This chapter has provided information about how your acupuncturist might diagnose and treat many common conditions. I have referred to named diseases in this chapter, as this is the way most of us understand our conditions. Your practitioner, although familiar with these terms, will also treat the underlying cause of your problem rather than dealing only with the named condition or the symptoms. If your condition is not included in this chapter your local practitioner will talk to you about whether acupuncture can help you.

10

Additional Treatment Methods: Auricular Acupuncture, Electro-acupuncture, Guasha and Cupping Therapy

In this chapter I'll look at some other, more unusual methods of treatment such as auricular acupuncture, electro-acupuncture and analgesia, guasha (scraping) therapy and cupping therapy.

Auricular acupuncture

What is auricular acupuncture?

Auricular acupuncture is a relatively new practice which utilises acupuncture points on the ear. It was developed in both China and France at around the same time. In 1956 Dr Paul Nogier, an acupuncturist and neurosurgeon, reported his experiences of auricular acupuncture at a congress in

Marseille and described using it to treat many conditions. Nogier had noticed that patients recovered from sciatic nerve pain when a nearby healer cauterised the anti helix, an area near the top of the ear. He was so fascinated by this discovery that he carried out research to find out if treating the ear could have other effects. This led him to continue until he had mapped the whole ear.

At around the same time some Chinese acupuncture practitioners were also finding out about the effectiveness of auricular acupuncture. Both Nogier and the Chinese practitioners discovered that points on the ear correspond to different parts of the body. The lobe of the ear, for example, corresponds to areas on the head, the inside of the ear to the internal organs of the body such as the Liver, Spleen, Stomach and Lungs and the outer ear to the upper and lower limbs.

What conditions does auricular acupuncture treat?

Auricular acupuncture is a complete system of treatment in itself. A few acupuncturists use it exclusively but most employ it in conjunction with treatment using acupuncture points on the body. Auricular acupuncture can treat many conditions both acute and chronic; it is especially beneficial for pain, particularly joint pain, and has become known for treating stomach, chest, intestinal, urinary, gynaecological and sinus problems. It can treat allergic conditions and inflammation and can be a great support for people who wish to stop smoking.

It can be helpful during childbirth. In this case treatment can calm the mother as well as alleviating pain. It is also well known for its use in the treatment of drug dependency. Childbirth and drug dependency treatments are described in more detail in Chapter 12.

Mike's anti-smoking treatment

Many people have experienced the beneficial effects of ear acupuncture in stopping smoking. In most cases it relieves the cravings and helps them to relax and adjust to being a non-smoker. Mike's results were exceptional, however, and he stopped wanting to smoke as soon as he had his first treatment. Mike is 71 years old. He had been smoking 40 cigarettes a day for 40 years when he went to see one of my colleagues over ten years ago. He had tried everything, including will-power, hypnosis and chewing gum, but nothing had worked. His doctor suggested acupuncture. Mike told me, 'The acupuncturist asked me: "Do you really want to give up?" and I said, "Yes I do." I was aware you have to be well motivated.' Mike finished his last cigarette before he went in for treatment. When he came out an hour later he no longer wanted to smoke. He told me, 'I had a full unopened pack in my car that remained there until I sold the car seven years later!' Mike had seeds attached to his ear that he could press if he felt cravings arise but rarely had to use them, finding that a dozen deep breaths were enough. He said, 'I still go to my acupuncturist every three to four months for a general tune up. My health is very good as a result and I haven't had a cold for years.'

How is auricular acupuncture carried out?

Before you are treated with auricular acupuncture your practitioner will both observe your ear and carefully examine it for areas of tenderness using a blunt probe. The tender areas indicate where in the body problems lie. Needles can then be inserted into these points, or small seeds or beads attached to them, in order to treat the areas that are imbalanced.

Different points have different effects. For example, a point in the triangular fossa, which is near the top of the earlobe, can be used if you are distressed or anxious and is very relaxing. Another point on the earlobe is called the 'eye' point. This corresponds with the point most commonly pierced if you wear

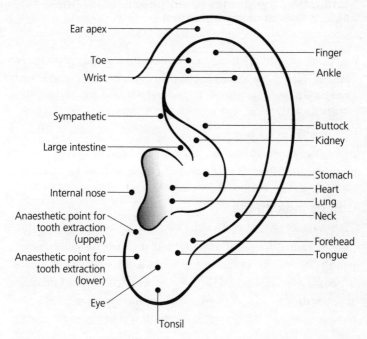

Map of the ear showing some of the acupuncture points

earrings. Gypsy travellers, who traditionally carried out the piercing of ears, positioned this point very precisely, as they knew that it benefited the eyesight.

There are points for your upper and lower limbs and points corresponding to all of your internal Organs, including the Lungs, Spleen, Kidneys, Heart and Liver. There are also points to relax your muscles, lower blood pressure, stop wheezing and clear the nose.

Stimulating the points using needles and press seeds

As I stated earlier, points are stimulated with either needles or tiny beads or seeds. During an acupuncture session, ear points are often needled at the same time as other points on the body. Seeds or beads can then usually be left in place after the treatment. The beads are securely fastened on to the ear with tape and you can stimulate them by pressing on the point. This gives a continued effect after the treatment is finished. These can be especially useful in the treatment of pain and addictions, or to aid relaxation.

Contra-indications

There are very few contra-indications for auricular acupuncture. Acupuncturists will take particular care with older people, young children and pregnant women. They will also be careful if people are weak, tired, hungry or anaemic. Alongside other acupuncture treatment, auricular acupuncture has been found to be a very safe and effective method of treatment.

Electro-acupuncture

What is electro-acupuncture?

Electro-acupuncture can sometimes be combined with auricular acupuncture. It is the stimulation of acupuncture points by an electrical current. A small hand-held, battery-operated machine about five inches long, four inches wide and one inch high is connected to the acupuncture needles via leads which clip on to them. The leads are plugged into output sockets and stimulation is controlled by means of dials on the machine. After the machine has been turned on the patient often controls the amount of stimulation going to the needles.

Using electro-acupuncture

I most frequently use electro-acupuncture if a patient has a 'full' as opposed to an 'empty' condition, especially when the patient has a lot of pain. It can be extremely effective for many of these conditions because it strongly clears through your channels when there is a blockage. Usually I treat patients experiencing a painful condition with ordinary acupuncture first. If the problem isn't responding and the patient is in extreme pain I might then consider using electro-acupuncture.

Some practitioners use this treatment more often than others. It can be used for pain relief during labour, for example, and it is also frequently used to treat hemiplegia (one-sided paralysis) following strokes as well as muscle spasms, inflammation, nerve damage and extreme joint pain. Some practitioners use it in conjunction with ear points to support a person going through withdrawal symptoms when stopping smoking or coming off drugs. It can be used for circulatory problems as well as to calm and relax people.

Sensations experienced during electro-acupuncture

When the needles are initially inserted into the points the sensation is the same as in ordinary treatment. The voltage of the electrical current is then slowly turned up until you feel a slight tingle around the point or along the energy pathway. This sensation is never stronger than is tolerable. The muscles may twitch a little bit but this is always kept to a comfortable level too.

How long are the needles left in?

The needles are left in for as long as you need them. This is usually 20 to 30 minutes. If a condition is extremely painful, for instance when a kidney stone is being passed or when a gallstone is causing obstruction, then they may be left in for longer.

How effective is electro-acupuncture?

Treatment is very effective for many of the conditions I have described above. Because it gives very strong stimulation it is not effective if you have a 'deficient' condition.

Contra-indications

Electro–acupuncture is contra–indicated for patients who have cancer, who are in a coma and in the first three months of pregnancy as well as for weak or frail patients.

Paul's electro-acupuncture treatment

Paul is 29 and works in the transport industry. He has had acupuncture for just over a year and now uses it preventatively, mainly to maintain his health and balance his moods. He has also had electro-acupuncture. 'I had an ankle injury that didn't get better. Two people literally stood on it in heavy boots during a football game. It was very painful and although the swelling had gone the pain remained. One of the treatments that helped it was electro-acupuncture.' He also has electro-acupuncture for a temporal mandibular joint (TMJ) problem which he has had for four years. He told me, 'I had visited many physiotherapists before discovering electro-acupuncture. I find it enormously helpful and would recommend it to anyone with this condition. I can literally feel the tension melt away when the area is stimulated. It is really the only thing that will deal with it and I'd be in an awful lot of pain if I didn't have it.'

Electro-acupuncture for analgesia

Acupuncture analgesia (pain relief) is carried out using electro-acupuncture and it has been used in China since the 1950s.

When I was in China in 1980 I saw two patients successfully having their thyroid removed and one having a heart operation using acupuncture as the sole anaesthetic. I still have photos of a patient waving to those of us watching while his operation was performed.

Acupuncture analgesia is carried out using the same small electro-acupuncture machine to stimulate the points. The electrical current which stimulates the needles is turned up slightly higher until it comfortably numbs the area which is to be operated on. Ear points or points on channels close to the area to be affected are used.

This form of analgesia can be extremely effective for certain conditions, especially those on the upper half of the body. It is an extremely safe for frail or elderly people, entailing less risk and a better recovery time than conventional anaesthetics. If it were used more extensively in the future it could help to cut down on the cost of the expensive anaesthetics that are currently used.

We may have a long wait before acupuncture analgesia is used on a large scale in Great Britain. Most acupuncturists do not specialise in this kind of treatment and tend to work in their own private practices. There is a growing trend, however, for acupuncturists to work in GPs' practices. As more professional acupuncturists begin to work in the National Health Service this treatment may gain in popularity.

Guasha therapy

Guasha is a treatment that goes back to at least the seventh century AD and has been passed down through Chinese families since that time. The word *gua* means 'to scrape' and *sha* means 'a rash' or 'spots like measles'. Guasha is carried out by scraping the surface of the skin with a smooth-edged, flat object until spots or other marks appear. Although guasha is a rather unusual treatment it can be a very effective way of treating many conditions.

The original uses of guasha

Guasha was originally used to treat colds and flu as well as to maintain good health. Traditionally many elderly people in China used it for health maintenance. The whole family knew how to carry out this therapy and younger members would use it to treat and maintain the health of the older generation. At one time the skin was scraped with a metal coin. Today a purpose-made flat scraper is employed. During the 1990s guasha suddenly became very popular in China and since then it has been developed to treat many more diseases.

What illnesses does guasha treat?

Guasha stimulates your Qi and Blood and can therefore be used to treat any condition where there is Qi and Blood stagnation, or to clear pathogens, especially Wind, Cold or Heat. As I explained above, guasha is particularly effective in treating colds and flu and for health maintenance but it can also be used for joint conditions such as shoulder, back, knee or neck problems. Other problems for which it has been used include asthma, bronchitis, headaches, high blood pressure, loose bowels, insomnia and post-viral syndromes.

How guasha is carried out

You will usually lie down on a couch to receive this treatment. Oil will then be lightly massaged on to your skin to provide a smooth surface. Any massage oil can be used although some practitioners may use special oils that contain herbs with additional Blood-moving qualities.

Scraping is always carried out by moving the blunt 'scraper' from top to bottom and from inside to outside. The therapy is never painful and your practitioner will check to ensure that you are comfortable while it is carried out.

The 'sha' or rash that appears when the skin is scraped indicates that Qi and Blood stagnation are being released from your body. Sometimes the sha is a light red colour, sometimes it is darker or even purple. Some people's skin may show more sha than others. Whatever the colour of the sha, the fact that it has appeared is always a positive sign. Sometimes no sha comes up when the skin is scraped. This usually indicates that there is no stagnation to be released.

How long does the sha last?

The sha will last for three to seven days and can look quite unsightly for a short time. Please note! Do not have this treatment before you are due to wear a low-cut ball gown or are about to go sunbathing on the beach. Occasionally the sha lasts longer than a week but it will always eventually fade. The next treatment on the area can be carried out after the sha from the previous treatment has disappeared. With each following treatment less and less sha will appear.

How much treatment will you need?

In general you will need one or two treatments for a cold or flu. Acute joint problems will also usually heal fairly quickly. More chronic problems can take longer and the number of treatments depends on your condition and how long you've had it. Guasha can be used as a long-term treatment if you are using it for health maintenance. The treatment is very safe and can be carried out on people who don't want to have needles.

Eva's guasha treatment

Although Eva is 65 she is still a very vital woman. She had her right arm amputated when she was only 19 because of cancer but has not let it affect her. She explained, 'A lot of muscles didn't work on that side but I've still run a business and brought up children, so the other arm does twice the work. Because of this it was very painful.'

Guasha combined with acupuncture has eased it. Her practitioner, a colleague, has used guasha on her neck, her shoulder and the base of her thumb, which are now much better. He has also treated the amputated side. Eva told me, 'Before treatment I couldn't bear to touch the area as it was too painful. Now it is no problem. I've had guasha only three times. My practitioner put oil on the area then used the guasha treatment before using acupuncture. The guasha was a bit painful. But it's definitely worth it, as its effects have been long term.'

Cupping therapy

Cupping is another popular treatment. It originated in China and is still used in many parts of Europe including Turkey, Greece, France and Italy. It removes Wind, Cold or Damp (see Chapter 5) that is trapped in the body and, like guasha, helps Qi or Blood that is 'stagnant' or not moving to flow freely again. Like guasha it temporarily leaves a red or purple mark on the skin. This is a good sign and it indicates that a pathogen is clearing from the body.

The cups in China are often made from bamboo. Bamboo cups are sometimes used in the West too, although most practitioners prefer glass cups.

What conditions might cupping be used for?

Cupping will often be used if you have joint problems such as swollen, painful or stiff joints, and it is also commonly used to clear a head cold.

How cupping is carried out

When each cup is applied a vacuum is first created inside it by placing a lighted taper quickly in the cup and removing it. The cup is then placed in position. The vacuum inside the cup creates suction and gently draws Qi and Blood to the surface allowing the release of any blocked pathogens. You will not feel any discomfort when this technique is used. As one of my patients said, 'When I saw the cups I thought they looked a bit strange. When they were actually in place I hardly noticed them, only a slight feeling of suction.' If cups are used to clear a common cold I tell the patient to wrap up warmly after the cups have been removed. The patient will then sweat and release Cold from her or his body.

Sometimes the cups are left in one position, at other times they may be moved. If moving cupping is used, oil is applied to the skin and the cups are moved over an area such as the back or shoulders. This can be very relaxing, as well as clearing blockages in the Qi.

Is it safe?

Yes, as long as it is used by a fully qualified practitioner. Because a lighted taper is used when carrying out the treatment, the practitioner is trained to ensure that she or he performs the technique safely. To eliminate risk, some practitioners prefer to use cups with suction pumps rather than creating a vacuum with a flame.

Anne's cupping treatment

Anne is 33 and works as an IT consultant. From the age of 12 her hands and feet were freezing cold even in mid-summer. Cupping carried out by one of my colleagues has changed this. She told me, 'I was constantly wearing fleeces and my friends would all take the mickey! I initially went to see my practitioner for stress and acupuncture quickly relaxed me. My practitioner then did cupping on my back. After two sessions I noticed that my hands weren't cold any more.' Anne had a thick white coating on her tongue, which had indicated to her practitioner that she had stagnation of Cold in her channels. As the cupping continued the tongue coating also disappeared. Anne didn't mind the cups, saying she only felt them creating a 'tight feeling' – although they did leave purple marks that took some days to disappear. It was worth it for the change they created. She told me, 'When I go to bed now I feel much warmer. It used to take me two to three hours to get warm and I would use a double duvet, an electric blanket and a hot water bottle as well as thick socks and thick fleecy pyjamas! I also had a cold and an ear infection recently and cupping sorted this out straight away – in fact as soon as I'd had the cupping I could breathe again. Cupping and acupuncture have changed my life significantly.'

Summary

- Auricular acupuncture, electro-acupuncture, guasha and cupping therapy are all treatments that are used by acupuncturists either instead of, or alongside, acupuncture treatment on the body.
- Auricular acupuncture involves placing small needles in the ear or attaching small seeds or beads to it. It can be used for acute or chronic conditions and is commonly used for pain, addictions and many other conditions.
- Electro-acupuncture is the stimulation of acupuncture points using an electric current. It is used to clear 'full' rather than 'deficient' conditions and is very helpful for extreme pain.

- Electro-acupuncture can be very effective when used to numb sensation for acupuncture analgesia – such as when carrying out an operation – or for pain relief.
- Guasha is scraping therapy. It is especially helpful to clear colds and flu and for health maintenance, although it can treat many other diseases.
- Cupping therapy is carried out by applying glass or bamboo cups to the body to draw out pathogens such as Wind, Cold or Damp. It can be beneficial for colds and flu and can also be used to treat many joint problems.

11

Children and Acupuncture

In China, many families bring their babies and children for acupuncture if they are ill. When I was doing clinical work in a hospital in China I would often be stunned to see the whole family come in with a child. Families knew how effective the treatment could be and they all wanted to give their support.

Here in the West children's acupuncture is a speciality that is becoming increasingly popular. Treatment in childhood can make the difference between a lifetime of health and a lifetime of illness, so treating children can be very gratifying for both the child and its parents.[1]

Children's illnesses

Common complaints treated in children

The most common conditions in children treated by acupuncture are coughs, asthma and glue ear. The list of conditions that it can treat, however, is far longer. For example, children respond really well to treatment for acute conditions such as colds and flu, as well as other infections such as tonsillitis, mumps and measles. Many of the digestive disorders that are frequently found in young children can be treated, as can common complaints such as respiratory conditions, insomnia, bowel problems, bed-wetting and epilepsy. Acupuncture is excellent for treating febrile convulsions – in China it is often the first treatment used when they occur. It is also one of the best treatments for cerebral palsy.

David's treatment

David has severe cerebral palsy and was treated with acupuncture by a colleague of mine for about four years. His mother once asked a physiotherapist to gauge how severely he was affected on a scale of 1 to 10. She said if 10 was the worst case she'd seen, he was about 8. Although acupuncture didn't cure all of his problems, it helped him tremendously.

One way in which treatment was stunningly successful was in the treatment of his eyes. He had a squint and eyes that rolled back. After one particular treatment his eyes came down and he was able to focus. They never reverted to their previous condition. He was also helped with the control of his head movements and he surprisingly never developed the chest problems that are usually found in children with cerebral palsy. The professionals would often ask his mother, 'Why hasn't he got a bad chest like other cerebral palsy children?' and she'd always answer, 'It's because of acupuncture.'

The treatment didn't help his constipation and although it had some effect on his spasms it didn't clear those completely either. His mother nevertheless said, 'I think that having the treatment made it possible for me to keep him from having the drugs which would normally be given to children with cerebral palsy. This meant that he was able to develop unusually good cognitive function. He could also follow instructions and do school work and I'm pleased to say that he knows where he is, who he is and will try to do lots of things. For these reasons alone treatment was worthwhile.'

Common illnesses that appear at different ages

Many children's illnesses that are treated with acupuncture occur at specific ages. For example, because of the fragility of the digestive system, it is common for children under six months old to have digestive complaints such as colic or diarrhoea. These frequently arise if the Organs become too cold or if milk and food starts accumulating in the digestive system. Such conditions often start shortly after birth, or when the child is being weaned and is adapting to new foods. Sometimes, if children are given a certain food before the digestive system can cope with it, they will become sensitive to that food or will develop other digestive problems later on in life. Acupuncture can sometimes prevent this from occurring.

At around two years old children are prone to develop fevers and other febrile diseases. Often these will be transitory and nothing to worry about. However, if more serious fevers and infections such as measles, whooping cough or mumps appear they can often be helped by acupuncture. Other conditions such as asthma, coughs, catarrh, sleep problems or glue ear may also arise at this age, while bed-wetting can be a problem after a child has been potty-trained.

After seven years children start to become aware of their own emotions. At this stage more obvious emotional problems, such as anxiety about schoolwork and exams, or about friendships, may develop and need to be treated. Children can have emotional problems before the age of seven, of course, but these are usually caused by parents not understanding the child's needs or the child reacting to stress in its environment. Many children can 'pick up' strong emotions around them and may react to their parents' difficulties and other strains. The appearance of a new sibling can also cause upheavals, of course, and jealousy can be a common trigger for some complaints.

Lifestyle is an increasingly common cause of illness in children and lack of exercise, poor diet, too much TV or staying up too late may all cause problems.

Treating children with acupuncture

At what age can children be treated?

Children of all ages can be treated. According to a colleague who runs a busy children's clinic, the largest number of children have treatment between the ages of two and four years, although he sees many older children too. He sees fewer children who are under one year old, although they too can benefit from treatment.

Diagnosing children

Observation plays a large part in the diagnosis of children and the practitioner will observe the child's behaviour, look and spirit. Palpation can be important too: the practitioner will notice the child's muscle tone and temperature as well as how the child deals with physical contact. Although pulse and tongue diagnosis is used on children over the age of four to five years, it is less reliable on younger children.

Children's responses to treatment

A child's energy tends to change much more rapidly than an adult's. This is partly because children don't have the same history of illness as adults or the same ongoing life problems. For example, they don't have to pay the mortgage or deal with complicated relationships – or bring up the children! Because they come with a 'clean slate' it is often possible to achieve long-lasting results in only a few treatments. There are exceptions, but children usually respond to treatment extremely quickly.

How do children deal with needles?

Using needles on children requires skill on the part of the practitioner, who will strive to introduce them in a way that doesn't upset the child. The child won't see the needles. Although half an hour of preparatory time might be needed so that the child is relaxed and ready for treatment, the whole process of using the needles will probably take no more than about two or three minutes. The needles are not left in. Children will often sit comfortably on their mother's lap while having treatment. In fact children are usually unperturbed at the end of the session and equally happy to come back for more treatment.

A few children are very scared of having needles and don't deal with them well. Usually this is caused by a Kidney deficiency, which, as you may remember, is associated with fear. In this case the child can have moxibustion treatment instead and this is usually effective.

Robin's asthma treatment

Robin is now 15 years old and he first had acupuncture when he was 13. Robin was diagnosed as having asthma when he was two and a half years old. He'd never suffered badly but he was allergic to dog hair and if he caught a cold it would go to his chest. He was prescribed some medication and later on used an inhaler if he needed it.

When Robin was 11 his mother took him to a doctor who pushed very hard for him to be given a cortisone-based drug. The doctor went as far as to say that if he didn't have the drug he would develop a heart problem and his growth would be stunted. The doctor wanted Robin to use the inhaler every day to get the drug into his system. His mother refused to give him this treatment, so he continued on Ventolin when he needed it. When he was 13 years old she took him to an acupuncturist. She told me, 'I think it was at exactly the right time and it has had an extremely positive effect. His chest has been so much better and he no longer takes inhalers at all.' He initially had three treatments and had a few boosters later; for example, he had treatment just before recent exams. While normally he would be a worrier, he coped with the exams incredibly well and was very relaxed.

This is what Robin says he experienced from treatment: 'I'm very sporty and always used to feel very tight-chested after distance runs or playing sports. Treatment has allowed me to breathe more freely and I'm now able to do sports without being overwhelmed by them. I can play football three or four times a week now with no trouble.'

How is children's acupuncture different from acupuncture for adults?

David and Robin had chronic conditions but children can be treated for acute conditions too. Children's illnesses such as infections, chest problems and convulsions often develop more swiftly than adult illnesses and can quickly become more serious. Because of this it is important that children get immediate treatment.

Children's illnesses are often related to the digestion. As I discussed above, Chinese medicine understands that a child's digestive system is more delicate than an adult's and hence they can only take food that is easily assimilated, such as milk. The digestive system can easily become strained, causing food to accumulate.

Children, like adults, can be strongly affected by emotional stresses. For some children these strains can have negative consequences for the rest of their life. If treatment changes the impact of these stresses it can have a profound effect on the child's future. As one practitioner told me, 'The difference between treating children and adults is rather like the difference between a light lace doily and heavy worsted fabric. Children's energy is so light and moves so easily that changes can be profound. It's rewarding to put the child's health back to where it should be – something has been invested in the child's future, in the very weave of the fabric.'

Finally, fewer needles are needed to treat a child than an adult. A young child often needs only two to four needles for the required effect to be achieved. The needles are not retained in a child as they sometimes are when an adult is treated.

Treating children is a worthwhile experience for those acupuncturists who specialise in this field. As another acupuncturist said, 'What could be more fulfilling than investing in the health of the next generation?'

Summary

- Children's illnesses are different from those of adults. In the West children's acupuncture is an increasingly popular speciality.
- Acupuncture treatment during childhood can make a huge difference to a child's future health.
- Children can be treated for a wide range of acute and chronic conditions.
- Children tend to respond more quickly than adults to acupuncture and often need fewer treatments.

12

Specialised Uses of Acupuncture: Childbirth, Drug Dependency, Animals and Facial Rejuvenation

Although acupuncture is over 2,000 years old, new methods of treatment are continually being developed. In this chapter I'll discuss some recent and specialised uses of treatment that are now very popular. These include treatment during pregnancy and labour, treatment for drug dependency, veterinary acupuncture and treatment for facial rejuvenation.

Treatment in pregnancy and childbirth

Pre- and post-natal treatment

I love attending births and feel a renewed sense of wonder and privilege whenever a new baby comes into the world – especially if it is with the help of acupuncture. As well as assisting during labour, acupuncture can also be used successfully for a variety of other situations in both pre- and post-natal care. For example, if you are pregnant, acupuncture can be used to induce labour if it is late or to turn a baby in a breech position. During labour it can be used for pain relief or to move labour forward if contractions slow down or stop. You can then be treated post-natally if you become depressed or depleted in energy.

Because the arrival of a baby is unpredictable not all acupuncturists are able to attend a birth. Many practitioners with busy practices find it difficult being on call while awaiting a birth because of the disruption it can cause. If you are pregnant and want to be helped by acupuncture, it is worth asking if your local practitioner is trained to assist with a birth. An increasing number of midwives are now training to become acupuncturists and it is also worth asking at your local maternity unit whether a qualified practitioner is available or can be recommended.[1]

Treatment for breech babies

Acupuncture to turn breech babies is increasingly popular and is often recommended at maternity units as a first choice of treatment. It is a very simple procedure for your acupuncturist to carry out and its success rate has been well established via research.

One study was carried out in Croatia on 67 pregnant women. They were all at least 34 weeks pregnant and all had a malpositioned or 'breech' baby. Half of the group were treated with acupuncture – a point at the end of the little toe was stimulated. The other 33 did not have any acupuncture treatment. Of those treated a stunning 76.4 per cent (26 women) were corrected, while of those not treated the babies of only 45.4 per cent (15 women) spontaneously turned. This treatment is both effective and relatively simple to carry out.[2]

Pain relief in labour

Acupuncture for pain relief in labour is more effective than gas and air. It is important to stress, however, that it is analgesia (pain relief) not anaesthesia (numbing the pain). As well as pain relief, the benefits of treatment during labour come in all sorts of other ways. For example, it can diminish fear as well as strengthening the mother's energy and increasing her sense of well-being. It can be especially useful during 'transition' in labour, which is the most difficult stage and when the mother becomes at her most distraught and unhappy.

Pain relief in childbirth is very beneficial because the reduced pain results in speedier and more efficient labour and cuts down the need for intervention. This doesn't mean that outside help is not needed at times, however – the results of acupuncture can be classified as varying from being extremely helpful to simply taking the edge off the pain and allowing you to deal with the labour better.

Research into acupuncture and pain relief in childbirth

A study carried out in Sweden found that women who received acupuncture during labour managed their labours with considerably less pain. It compared 90 women who had acupuncture with 90 who did not. Fifty-two of the women (58 per cent) who had acupuncture managed their deliveries without further pain treatment compared with only 13 (14 per cent) who didn't have acupuncture. Ninety-four per cent of the patients who had acupuncture said they would consider having acupuncture again during future deliveries. The authors concluded that acupuncture reduces the need for other methods of pain relief in childbirth.[3]

Where will the needles be placed?

Needles for pain relief will be placed in points in the upper and lower limbs and the lower back. The points chosen will vary according to your needs. Points on the ear may also be used very successfully. Auricular points include ones for the pelvis, for the endocrine system and for the uterus, as well as calming and relaxing points. Some practitioners use these ear points with a hand-held electro-acupuncture machine that can be controlled by the patient. She can then ensure that the stimulation is at the correct level to relieve the pain.

Induction

Acupuncture is often used to induce birth if the baby is over-due. A mother-to-be usually goes to an acupuncturist if she does not want to be chemically induced. The acupuncturist will treat by stimulating a number of points. One of these lies on the Spleen channel on the inside lower leg. Treating this point has a direct effect on the uterus and can start to stimulate contractions.

Morning sickness

Morning sickness can be extremely disabling and acupuncture can be very helpful. The nausea may have a number of different causes. For instance, Phlegm may be blocking the Stomach, the Stomach and Spleen Qi may be deficient or there may be a disharmony between the Spleen and the Liver. Your acupuncturist will usually treat this condition using points on both your legs and arms. For example, one point that is commonly used is about a quarter of the way up the inside of the arm. This point not only deals with morning sickness but can also be used to treat any kind of nausea and vomiting. Because of its usefulness, this is the point used for 'sea bands', which are bands that can be attached to the wrist to help people with sea sickness.

Post-natal depression and exhaustion

Finally, it has already been mentioned in Chapter 10 that acupuncture is used very successfully to treat depression. One common cause of post-natal depression is blood loss. Treatment to nourish the Blood can have an extremely beneficial effect on the mother. Many mothers find that acupuncture will calm and strengthen them after birth and that their babies are subsequently happier too. This creates a positive cycle with each becoming calmer and happier and more able to cope well.

Sandra's acupuncture treatment to induce labour

When Sandra's baby was one week overdue she turned to acupuncture for help. She told me, 'The consultant broke my waters and then told me I had two hours to go into labour or I would be induced. I immediately phoned my acupuncturist, as I had no contractions. Two minutes after my practitioner put needles in me the contractions started. Even my husband, who is very sceptical, noticed that it was quite obvious that the acupuncture changed things immediately.' Her practitioner went on to give her pain relief during the labour and although she has no way of knowing how painful it would have been without the acupuncture, the labour was very bearable and she didn't take any drugs. Sandra now says, 'If I have another baby I'd definitely have acupuncture again.'

Auricular acupuncture and treatment for drug dependency

Another more recent use of acupuncture is as a treatment for those who are dependent on drugs. As problems of drug

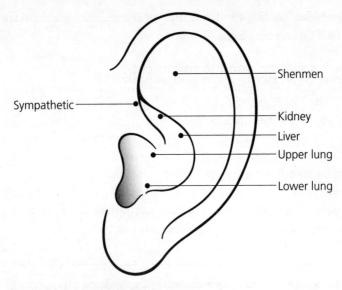

Shenmen

Sympathetic

Kidney
Liver
Upper lung

Lower lung

The five 'detox' points
(Please note: *either* Upper lung *or* Lower lung would be used.)

dependency and alcohol abuse continue to grow, auricular acupuncture stands out as one successful method of achieving withdrawal. This treatment was first used in the early 1970s and it is now employed extensively throughout the Western world.

To carry out the treatment five main points on the ear are used and these help to detoxify the body. While the needles are in place the patient relaxes for up to 45 minutes listening to quiet music. The points help to reduce the pain of withdrawal, including such effects as vomiting, cramps, sweats and pains in the joints. They also reduce the craving for drugs. When people are withdrawing from drugs they are often jumpy and aggressive; this treatment calms their energy and settles them down.

Very often people who have come in agitated will relax and fall asleep during treatment.

Drugs that respond to treatment

Auricular acupuncture was first used on methadone users. It was then found to be useful for cocaine, crack cocaine, ecstasy, heroin and many other drugs as well as prescription drugs like Valium. It is also used for alcohol abuse.

Coming for treatment

If people are withdrawing from drugs they have treatment every day if possible. Drug rehabilitation units are usually run on a 'drop-in' basis and provide a group situation that is a supportive environment for people coming off drugs by means of acupuncture.

Drug users often start by having only auricular acupuncture in the drop-in group. After about six treatments they might combine this with one-to-one acupuncture that is directed more towards their individual problems. In some drug rehabilitation centres acupuncture is used in combination with counselling provided by the centre.

Clearing drugs from the body

Opiates such as heroin can be cleared out of the system in as little as two to three days, or at most up to two weeks. Methadone is much harder and takes longer. Cannabis stays in the system for about one month and tranquillisers are the hardest to deal with, taking from 12 to 18 months to completely disappear from the body.

Staying off drugs

Results from this treatment vary according to the individual being treated, which drugs they are taking and how motivated they are to stop. In a follow-up survey carried out by a centre in Brighton it was found that of 94 people who had a combination of auricular acupuncture and one-to-one treatment, most had reduced stress and anxiety and an improvement in their energy, mood and ability to sleep. Of these people, those who came off alcohol fared the best, but people also succeeded in coming off prescription drugs, giving up smoking and coming off other recreational or street drugs.

How well this treatment works over a long period of time has not yet been established but I am told by acupuncturists in this field that it is now a mainstream therapy which is used in all drug rehabilitation centres in Greater London and in most other parts of the UK. This in itself is a testimony to its efficacy.

The problem of drug abuse is unfortunately on the increase. This treatment is one successful way of assisting patients with the problem.

Tom's auricular acupuncture treatment

Tom's acupuncture has helped him to come off drugs. When he talked to me he'd had treatment for only nine weeks and had already noticed that it had made a difference in many ways. He is 46 years old and is married with two children. He told me, 'I have ear acupuncture four days a week. It is amazingly helpful. In fact I'd now rather have needles than take a pill! Before having treatment I was on eighty milligrams of methadone as well as Diazepam and cannabis. After nine weeks I had cut down to twenty milligrams of methadone. I had stopped taking the Diazepam altogether after the third or fourth ear acupuncture session. I still smoke cannabis occasionally.'

Tom has a long history of drug taking. He started smoking cannabis as a teenager, then joined the army where he took Dexedrine and Benzedrine. After leaving the army he went into the music business, and he describes his life from then on as 'sex, drugs and rock and roll' all the way. He was on heroin for 14 or 15 years – an experiment which got out of hand – then went on to methadone as a substitute for heroin. He had been on a methadone programme for 18 months before having acupuncture.

'Recently I realised that I needed help and that's when I started the ear acupuncture. My wife and I both took drugs and we knew that we couldn't keep taking them. Now we have the children we have to clean up our act.'

As well as having ear acupuncture, Tom has one-to-one acupuncture treatment and this helps him to build up his emotional strength. 'At the moment my defences are low – I watch *Blue Peter* and want to burst into tears.' If he goes in for treatment feeling anxious, he feels relaxed and easy afterwards and it acts as a buffer for him. 'It's so interesting that I can have a needle in my toe and it helps me feel better. I've done very well so far and look forward to the day I come off drugs altogether.'

Veterinary acupuncture

How popular is veterinary treatment?

The popularity of veterinary acupuncture has mushroomed in the last ten years. As mainstream acupuncture becomes more available, people want their pets treated too. Its appeal has been helped in recent years by popular TV programmes such as *Vets in Practice* and *The Dog Whisperer*.

There is another reason for its popularity. In recent years pets have taken far greater priority in people's lives and are also living longer. During the later stages of their lives there are fewer conventional medicines to help them. People are happy to pay for treatments that keep their beloved pets healthy and acupuncture is one that can be of great help and support.

Which animals are commonly treated?

The animals most commonly brought to a veterinary acupuncturist are small pets such as dogs and cats. Some horses are also treated – in fact some equine vets specialise in using acupuncture. Sheep or cattle could be treated but rarely are, as acupuncture wouldn't be considered a cost-effective treatment for farm animals.

Do animals mind having needles?

I have it on good authority that animals don't mind having needles at all – in fact many will doze off when they have treatment. You might be surprised to know that this especially applies to cats. If a cat is wrapped securely in a blanket and feels safe it will be happy to have treatment and will often sleep afterwards. I am told that dogs are also easy to treat. They don't feel the needles at all because they have no nerve endings in their skin. Horses too respond well and instantly become calm when they are treated.

Common illnesses for which animals have treatment

The vast majority of animals are brought to treatment for joint problems and pain conditions. These include conditions such as arthritis, back pain (including disc problems), hip problems, injuries involving ligaments, tendons and muscles, and paralysis. Acupuncture can also be used for bowel and digestive conditions and for sinus problems and catarrh.

The results of veterinary acupuncture

Just like humans, each animal responds to treatment in its own unique way. As a general rule, however, animals' responses to treatment fall into three main groups.

The first group responds strongly and well from the very first treatment onwards.

The second, and by far the largest, group shows a slightly slower improvement. They initially need to come for treatment once a week. By the third treatment they are usually showing signs of improvement. For example, a dog may start to bark at the vacuum cleaner or be picking up its toys again. By the fourth treatment these energetic changes may be followed by more visible physical signs of improvement. As long as the animal continues to progress, after the sixth treatment the sessions may be spread out, becoming fortnightly or four-weekly. Later, if all goes well, they will take place three or four times a year.

Finally, a small sub-group of pets do not respond to treatment, but these are the exception rather than the rule.

The law and treating animals

In the UK acupuncture treatment on animals is considered to be a surgical act. It is illegal for anyone other than a vet to use acupuncture to treat animals – in fact it is easier to treat humans than animals![4] Veterinary nurses, however, may treat animals under the auspices of a veterinary surgeon. It is also legal for anyone to treat their own pet.

Some veterinary colleges now teach acupuncture as an adjunctive therapy in their curriculum and happily it is increasingly being seen as part of mainstream veterinary education. This is very good news both for animals and for their owners, who can more easily have their pets treated.

Shea's veterinary acupuncture treatment

Shea is a nine-year-old border collie who suffers from hip dysplasia and osteo-arthritis which started when he was three years old. His first symptoms were stiffness at night and a change in his walking. His legs then gave way under him. His owner took him to a vet who diagnosed the condition. When, one year later, it was getting worse she took him to a veterinary acupuncturist. Shea's owner told me, 'After the third treatment he started to change and became happier. I rang a friend and said, "I've got my dog back!" A couple of treatments after that I noticed his walking had improved. He was less stiff and he could go up and down stairs more easily. When he has a treatment Shea gets very sleepy and relaxed, then curls up and goes to sleep. Then he gets perky again and the vet says, "It's time to take the needles out." My original vet had discussed how Shea might have only a few years to live and how I would not be able to let him off a lead when he went for walks. He would have had no quality of life. He's now nine years old. I thought he'd never make it, but he has a good quality of life and his whole demeanour has also changed – I put it down to acupuncture.'

Acupuncture for facial rejuvenation

Facial rejuvenation is one of the newest acupuncture treatments being used in the West. With the popularity of other anti-ageing and anti-wrinkle treatments it is not surprising that it is fast becoming all the rage. When I first heard of this treatment a couple of years ago I must admit I rejected it outright. I said to myself, 'I'm not a beauty therapist, I'm here to treat sick people.' As time has gone on I've mellowed. Although I don't use it myself, I've now grown to accept that this is one of a range of potentially beneficial treatments and that it can sometimes be a person's first introduction to the deeper and more health-giving effects of acupuncture.

What does it do?

Facial rejuvenation is a technique that is used to improve the complexion, reduce lines on the face and improve muscle tone, which becomes lax as you age. It achieves this effect by locally invigorating the Qi and Blood. It encourages the Blood supply to the face, promotes lymph drainage and creates new cellular growth.

Who does it?

This technique should only be carried out by qualified professional acupuncturists who have had post-graduate training in the use of this procedure.

Who has it?

The majority of people who decide to come for this treatment are not surprisingly women, and most are in their mid to late forties. It is, of course, available to older or younger people and to men as well as women.

How is it done?

The methods used for carrying out facial rejuvenation vary slightly according to the practitioner. Some practitioners attach the needles to a small hand-held electro-acupuncture machine and others use needles without stimulation. Some practitioners use an electro-acupuncture machine with pads rather than needles, while others use massage on the face and employ needles on more distal points. Some use a combination of the different techniques.

If needles are used they will not penetrate deeply, only being inserted just under the surface of the skin. Clinics using facial treatments are now springing up all over China and are very popular. Practitioners in these clinics use both herbal and acupuncture treatments.

What kind of result might you expect?

The results gained from this treatment naturally depend entirely on the individual patients and the initial condition of their skin.

If a person eats well and is generally healthy it will often support the effects of the treatment. The results can range from no effect to dramatic changes and no acupuncturist using these techniques will make guarantees. The most common result of treatment is that other people start commenting, 'You look good today!'

How many treatments does each person have?

Acupuncturists tend to encourage those having treatment to commit themselves initially to at least six treatments. This is because results tend to be cumulative. After this time, if people feel happy with the effects they can either decide to stop or continue according to their needs. Most people have about 20 treatments and during this time they might also have more general treatment for their underlying health.

By the end of the treatments the person might expect to look in the mirror and feel good about themselves, and they should be benefiting from the holistic treatment too. Many people who have started treatment for facial rejuvenation continue to have acupuncture to maintain their general balance of health. Treatment is not necessarily going to be miraculous but it will help people to look brighter and fresher.

Is it safe?

It is completely safe as long as your practitioner is a professional acupuncturist trained in the use of this treatment. It can occasionally, but not always, leave mild bruising for a few days. This bruising is nothing like the bruising that results from botox or cosmetic surgery, of course, and there are no side effects at all.

Karen's facial rejuvenation

Karen is a busy 47-year-old designer who has had five treatments. Her acupuncturist was recommended by a friend who came back from treatment saying, 'I feel so young after it!' Karen decided that she needed some 'TLC' and thought she'd try it too. She went with an open mind but is now hooked. She told me, 'He stuck needles all over my face but I hardly felt them. After the first treatment the effect was the most dramatic. It was as if I couldn't frown any more. I could feel the muscles on the outer part of my forehead but not the inner part. It didn't last for the whole week, but now I've had five treatments I'm much less inclined to frown and the whole area is better – it's like natural botox. I also got very puffy under my eyes sometimes. That has completely gone too. It feels good to go for treatment, it's my treat and something just for me.'

Summary

- Acupuncture can be used during labour, as well as pre- and post-natally. It can be especially helpful for pain relief during labour, to turn breech babies, to induce babies who are overdue, to relieve morning sickness and for post-natal depression and exhaustion.

- Auricular acupuncture has been used since the 1970s to support people who are withdrawing from drugs. Five 'detox' points are used and while the needles are left in place the patient can relax and listen to quiet music. Some patients supplement this treatment with one-to-one acupuncture on the body.

- Veterinary acupuncture is an increasingly popular and effective treatment for pets, especially cats, dogs and horses. It can help with many conditions, particularly joint problems and pain.

- Acupuncture for facial rejuvenation is one of the newest acupuncture treatments in the West. It is used to improve the complexion, reduce fine lines and improve muscle tone.

13

Finding the Right Practitioner

You now have a good overview of acupuncture and its benefits. In this final chapter I will provide guidance on how to find a practitioner, how to decide if she or he is well qualified, how to assess if she or he is right for you and how you might work with your doctor when reducing any medication.

Finding a good practitioner

Most people find a practitioner by personal recommendation. For instance, Josie commented, 'A friend had benefited from treatment and said her practitioner was a caring and sensitive person. I wanted to get pregnant and I thought, "I want to try it."' Jenny was similar, telling me, 'A friend's mum had already gone to the clinic and told me I should go. I'd tried everything else really so I thought I'd try it.' Craig, Francesca and Sarah also had recommendations from either friends or family and Samantha from her GP. If you want to have acupuncture and know people who have had successful treatment, you can ask them for the name of their practitioner.

If you don't know of anyone in your area or if you have doubts about a practitioner's qualifications, then you can contact one of the professional bodies for acupuncture in your country. In the UK this is the British Acupuncture Council (BAcC). These professional bodies will gladly tell you who is practising in your area and ensure that you are recommended to an acupuncturist who is well trained.

Sometimes you may be faced with too much choice. If there are a large number of acupuncturists in your area then you may need to decide which one is best suited to you. If you don't have a recommendation then ask the practitioner of your choice to have a short chat to you about treatment. Many acupuncturists offer a free 15–20 minute chat. This will allow you to meet the acupuncturist, ask any questions and see the premises. If you then feel comfortable with the practitioner you can book an appointment.

Checking that your acupuncturist is well qualified

There are a number of ways for you to check that your acupuncturist is properly qualified. First ensure that your practitioner belongs to a professional body such as the British Acupuncture Council (see the Useful Addresses section of this book).

Second, find out about your practitioner's training. Most acupuncturists will have completed a three- or four-year course before qualifying. Some doctors and physiotherapists have done short weekend courses that are mainly aimed at relieving pain. Practitioners who have taken short courses are not well qualified as acupuncturists, even if they are first-rate practitioners in their own profession. Some doctors and physiotherapists have completed full training, so it is worth checking. A poorly qualified practitioner will not be able to achieve the same results with treatment as one who is well trained.

Third, make sure that she or he takes a thorough case history before starting treatment. No practitioner can treat you holistically without making a diagnosis first. A good practitioner will also feel the pulses on your wrist and look at your tongue.

Fourth, it is important to notice how you get on with your acupuncturist. Is she or he interested in you and do you have a good rapport? Do you like and trust this person?

When I talked to patients about treatment it was clear that they placed a high priority on their relationship. For example, Francesca told me, 'It was very important that I trusted my practitioner. I experienced her desire to help me and that she was on my side. She was also easy to get on with and our rapport was really good.' Craig said, 'My relationship with my practitioner was absolutely vital – it is a relationship of trust and understanding.'

Why is a professional body important?

A professional body will protect you as a member of the general public. It ensures that practitioners follow a code of practice and a code of ethics and uphold the highest standards of hygiene. All practitioner members of a professional body also carry insurance. As part of the above codes, practitioners will also, of course, keep anything you say in the treatment room confidential.

Going for treatment

Where do acupuncturists practise?

Most professional acupuncturists in the UK currently treat in private practices although a few treat in the National Health Service. Even if your practitioner works in the NHS it is still important to ensure that they have had a thorough training as a practitioner.

Many practitioners work in clinics. These can be acupuncture clinics that house a number of acupuncturists[1] or multi-disciplinary clinics where many types of practitioners work together in one practice. For example, in such a clinic herbalists, massage therapists, osteopaths and chiropractors may be working under one roof. Many practitioners now work from a GP's practice and some practise from their own homes. The standard of hygiene in your acupuncturist's premises is checked by an environmental health officer if you live in the UK. If you live in another country it too will have an equivalent person who ensures hygiene standards. Your acupuncturist follows stringent rules that have been laid down by his or her professional body.

Preparation before the treatment

No special preparation is needed before a treatment although it is best to arrive feeling as prepared as possible. It can be useful to make a note of what you want to talk to your acupuncturist about, just in case you forget. It can also be important not to have a heavy meal before treatment, but at the same time not to have no food at all.

Bring to the initial consultation a list of medicines you are taking and any relevant X-rays. This first session can sometimes take up to one and a half hours and subsequent treatments from half to one hour. The exact duration will vary from practitioner to practitioner, so it can be useful to check how long it will take and to allow enough time.

After the treatment

Ideally it is best to leave time after the treatment to relax and avoid any physical or mental stress. Your body, mind and spirit are making adjustments and relaxation will help the process. Try not to do anything extreme after a treatment, such as eating a huge meal, having an excessively hot bath or being strenuously active. If you have had your Liver Qi treated don't drink alcohol after treatment. Your Liver can become very sensitive and small amounts will then have a strong effect.

Should I tell my doctor that I'm having treatment?

You are not required to tell your doctor that you are having treatment although many people like to let their doctor know. Most doctors, though not all, will be comfortable that a patient is having acupuncture and some, like Samantha's, recommend it. Whether you tell your doctor or not depends on what you are being treated for. If you are taking prescribed drugs then it is best to inform her or him. The issue of coming off any drugs can then be addressed when relevant.

Prescribed drugs and acupuncture treatment

You will not need to come off your prescribed medication in order to have acupuncture treatment. As you become healthier through treatment, however, you may wish to cut down on any medication you are taking and if possible stop taking them. This depends on the medicines and why you are taking them.

Your acupuncturist is trained to understand the effects of medication and will advise you on this matter. If you wish to start reducing your drugs she or he will often ask you to consult your doctor and withdraw the medicines with the doctor's full support.

Some drugs can be cut down naturally. For example, patients will stop taking painkillers if they no longer have pain or will gradually cut down on sleeping pills as their sleep improves. Other medications cannot be withdrawn at all; for instance, some replacement drugs such as insulin for diabetics or vitamin B12 for patients with pernicious anaemia. If patients are unable to fully withdraw from some medicinal drugs, treatment can still help them to improve their health generally and cope better with their illness.

A final thought

The Chinese have a saying that 'good health is the root of happiness'. My personal experience of acupuncture bears this out. For those of you who have decided to have treatment, I hope this book has clarified the potential benefits and also dispelled some of the myths about acupuncture. I also hope that you are helped in at least as many ways as the patients who have featured in this book. Good luck to you on your journey to health and happiness.

Notes

Chapter 1

1   A. Vickers, P. Wilson, J. Kleijnen, *Quality and Safety in Health Care* (2002).

2   J. Shaw, P. Bidgood and N. Sacbi, 'Exploring Acupuncture Outcomes in a College Clinic. Patient Profile and Evaluation of Overall Treatment Benefit', *European Journal of Oriental Medicine*, Vol. 5(4), pp. 55–63.

3   R. Chapman, R. Norton, C. Paterson, 'A Descriptive Outcome Study of 291 Acupuncture Patients', *European Journal of Oriental Medicine*, Vol. 3(5) (2001), pp. 48–53.

4   W. Weidenhammer, A. Streng, K. Linde, A. Hoppe, D. Melchart, 'Acupuncture for Chronic Pain Within the Research Programme of 10 German Health Insurance Funds – Basic Results From an Observational Study', *Complementary Therapies in Medicine,* Vol. 15(4) (2006), pp. 238–246.

5   For more on Qi see Chapter 7.

6   The British Acupuncture Council (BAcC) gives the names of well trained acupuncturists. This is the largest professional body for acupuncturists in the UK. The address and website are listed at the end of the book.

7   Always check your practitioner's training. Professional acupuncturists who use the traditional style of treatment you will read about in this book have studied for at least three years in order to become competent practitioners. Some doctors and physiotherapists have taken short courses in acupuncture lasting only one or two weekends and do not use the underlying theory of Chinese medicine. These practitioners will usually be trained to deal with a limited range of conditions and are unlikely to be treating the

underlying cause of the patient's condition, as would a profes-sional practitioner.

8   World Health Organization, *Acupuncture Review and Analysis of Reports on Controlled Clinical Trials* (2003), pp. 9–10.

9   K.J. Sherman, R.R. Coeytaux, 'Acupuncture for Improving Chronic Back Pain, Osteoarthritis and Headache', *Journal of Clinical Outcomes Management*, Vol. 16(5) (2009), pp. 224–30.

10   E. Manheimer, S. Wieland, E. Kimbrough, K. Cheng, B.M Berman, 'Evidence from the Cochrane Collaboration for Traditional Chinese Medicine Therapies', *Journal of Alternative and Complementary Medicine*, Vol. 15(9) (2009), pp. 1001–14.

11   K.K. Hui, S. Hui, 'The Salient Characteristics of the Central Effects of Acupuncture Needling: Limbic-Paralimbic-Neocortical Network Modulation', *Human Brain Mapping*, Vol. 30(4) (2009), pp. 1196–206.

12   M. Beck, 'Decoding an Ancient Therapy: High-Tech Tools Show How Acupuncture Works in Treating Arthritis, Back Pain and Other Illnesses', *Wall Street Journal, Health Journal*, 22 March 2010.

13   S.J. Birch, R.L. Felt (1999) pp. 154–66.

Chapter 2

1   J. Shaw, P. Bidgood and N. Sacbi, 'Exploring Acupuncture Outcomes in a College Clinic. Patient Profile and Evaluation of Overall Treatment Benefit', *European Journal of Oriental Medicine*, Vol. 5(4), pp. 55–63.

2   This covers arthritis and joint pains.

3   J. Shaw, P. Bidgood and N. Sacbi, 'Exploring Acupuncture Outcomes in a College Clinic. Patient Profile and Evaluation of Overall Treatment Benefit', *European Journal of Oriental Medicine*, Vol. 5(4), pp. 55–63.

4   Fibro-myalgia is chronic, widespread pain in muscles and soft tis-sues surrounding joints, accompanied by fatigue.

5   B. Flaws, J. Lake, *Chinese Medicinal Psychiatry*, Blue Poppy Press, Boulder (Co), (2001).

6   Acute illnesses have a sudden onset and severe symptoms but usu-ally have a short duration.

7   World Health Organization, *Acupuncture Review and Analysis of Reports on Controlled Clinical Trials* (2003), pp. 9–10.

8   K.J. Sherman, R.R. Coeytaux, 'Acupuncture for Improving Chronic Back Pain, Osteoarthritis and Headache', *Journal of Clinical Outcomes Management*, Vol. 16(5) (2009), pp. 224–30.

9   World Health Organization, *Acupuncture Review and Analysis of Reports on Controlled Clinical Trials* (2003), pp. 9–10.

10   C.A. Smith, P.P. Hay, H. Macpherson, 'Acupuncture for Depression', *Cochrane Database System Review*, Vol. 20(1) (2010): CD004046.

11   M.S. Lee, B.C. Shin, P. Ronany, E. Ernst, Acupuncture for Schizophrenia: A Systematic Review and Meta-Analysis, *International Journal of Clinical Practice*, Vol. 63(11) (2009), pp. 1622–33.

12   P.M. Wayne, R. Hammerschlag, H.M. Langevin, V. Napadow, J.J. Park, R.N. Schnyer, 'Resolving Paradoxes in Acupuncture Research: A Roundtable Discussion', *Journal of Alternative Complementary Medicine*, Vol. 15(9) (2009), pp. 1039–44.

13   World Health Organization, *Acupuncture Review and Analysis of Reports on Controlled Clinical Trials* (2003), p. 14.

14   ME Stands for Myalgic Encephalomyelitis. 'Myalgic' means pain in the muscles and 'Encephalomyelitis' means inflammation of the brain and nerves. ME or Chronic Fatigue Syndrome (CFS) can appear gradually and insidiously without any apparent infection, or after an acute infection.

15   World Health Oraganization, *Acupuncture Review and Analysis of Reports on Controlled Clinical Trials* (2003), p. 12.

16   J.J Wang, Y.J Song, Z.C. Wu, X.O. Chu, X.H. Wang, X.J. Wang, L.N. Wei, Q.M. Wang, 'A Meta-Analysis on Randomized Controlled Trials of Acupuncture Treatment of Chronic Fatigue Syndrome', *Zhen Ci Yan Jiu*, Vol. 34(6) (2009), pp. 421–8.

17   S.K Kim, H. Bae, 'Acupuncture and Immune Modulation', *Autonomic Neuroscience*, April 2010 [epub ahead of print].

18   B. J. Anderson, F. Haimovici, E.S. Ginsburg, D.J. Schust, P.M. Wayne, 'In Vitro Fertilization and Acupuncture: Clinical Efficacy and Mechanisitic Basis', *Alternative Therapies In Health And Medicine*, Vol. 13(3) (2007), pp. 38–48.

19   'The Efficacy of Acupoint Stimulation for the Management of Therapy Related Adverse Events in Patients with Breast Cancer', *Breast Cancer Res Treat*, Vol. 118(2) (2009), pp. 255–67.

20   World Health Organization, *Acupuncture Review and Analysis of Reports on Controlled Clinical Trials* (2003), pp. 20–1.

21 E. Manheimer, G. Zhang, L. Udoff, A. Haramat, P. Langenbrg, B.M. Berman, L.M. Bouter, 'Effects of Acupuncture on Rates of Pregnancy and Live Birth Among Women Undergoing In Vitro Fertilisation: Systematic Review and Meta-Analysis', *British Medical Journal,*Vol. 336(7643) (2008), pp. 545–9.
22 World Health Organization, *Acupuncture Review and Analysis of Reports on Controlled Clinical Trials* (2003), p. 16–17.

Chapter 3

1 In the UK this is usually the British Acupuncture Council (BAcC). For a list of professional bodies in other countries see Useful Addresses at the end of this book.
2 When I was in China, I noticed that Chinese Patients were far better at distinguishing pain from sensation than patients in the West. Chinese patients use the word pronounced *suan* to indicate that they feel the sensation from the needle. This is different from the word that describes pain, however, which is *tong*. (There are fewer words in the English language to describe pain or sensation than in the Chinese language.)

Chapter 4

1 In the terminology of Western medicine the Pericardium is a smooth membranous sac that envelops the heart.
2 S. Hicks (1999), p. 21.

Chapter 5

1 N. Black, D. Boswell, G. Alastair, S. Murphy, J. Popay (1990).
2 The 1991 Census, HMSO (1993), Limiting Long-Term Illness for Great Britain, Title 3.
3 For more in-depth information on the causes of disease see A. Hicks (2001).
4 M. Gauquelin, *How Atmospheric Conditions Affect Your Health*, ASI Publishers Inc. 1989, p. 39.
5 Severe windy weather affecting our health has been well documented in many countries. Nations in Central Europe describe

fohn winds. North Americans describe *chinook* and *santa ana* winds. Israelis know when the *sharav* blows. Australians are aware of *Easterlies*, *Westerlies* or *Northerlies*. These winds are all said to cause problems varying from headaches and migraines to an increased incidence of accident, crime and suicide rates. See M. Kaiser, *How the Weather Affects Your Health*, Hill of Content, Michelle Anderson Publishing, Pty Ltd., Ch. 2, p. 26.

6   C. Peterson, M. Seligman, G. Vaillant, 'Pessimistic Explanatory Style is a Risk Factor for Physical Illness: A thirty-five-year longitudinal study', *Journal of Personality and Social Psychology*, Vol. 55(1) (1988), pp. 23–7.

7   Taken from A. Hicks (2010).

8   *Su Wen*, Ch. 39.

9   R.A. Nicholson, S.E. Gramling, J.C. Ong, L. Buenevar, *Headache*, Vol. 43(6), St Louis School of Medicine (2003), pp. 651–63.

10   T. Ohira, H. Iso, T. Tanigawa et al., *Journal of Hypertension*, Vol. 20(1), Institute of Community Medicine, University of Tsukuba, Japan (2002), pp. 21–7.

11   Research carried out by National Opinion Poll for *Bella*, November 1996.

12   Y.H. Zhang, K. Rose (1995), p. 73.

13   J. Li, D. Hansen, P.B. Mortensen, J. Olsen, *Circulation*, Vol. 106(13) (September 2002), pp. 1634–9.

14   D. Goleman (1995), p. 174.

15   Ibid., p. 100.

16   L. Breslow, N. Breslow, 'Health Practices and Disability: Some Evidence from Alameda County', *Preventative Medicine* (1993), pp. 86–95.

17   N. Armstrong, A. McManus, 'Children's Fitness and Physical Activity', *British Journal of Physical Education* (Spring 1994).

18   For more on the causes of disease see A. Hicks 2010.

Chapter 6

1   H. Lu (1973), Ch. 2.

2   Face reading is an art used in Chinese medicine for thousands of years. For more on face reading see L. Bridges (2004).

3   Many practitioners of Qigong (Chinese health exercises) say that regular practice of it will conserve Essence and can even build it up.

4   This refers to Damp that arises from the inside. Damp can also arise from the outside and this is described in Chapter 4.
5   This generally correlates with the condition known in Western medicine as manic depression or bipolar.

Chapter 7

1   All quotes from the *Su Wen* are taken from C. Larre and E. Rochat de Valle (1992).
2   Famously known as a 'malapropism' after Mrs Malaprop in the play *The Rivals* by Richard Brinsley Sheridan.
3   The nearest equivalent in Western medicine is the cerebral spinal fluid that lies in the spine and brain.
4   The famous serenity prayer states, 'God grant me the serenity to accept the things I cannot change, courage to change the things I can and the wisdom to know the difference.'
5   These Elements date back to the *Zhou* dynasty in China which is about 1000–750 BC.
6   For more on Five Element Acupuncture and the Constitutional Factor, see A. Hicks, J. Hicks and P. Mole, 2010.

Chapter 8

1   *Please do not expect them to be 100 per cent accurate* – questionnaires can never take the place of a diagnosis by your practitioner.
2   For more on menopausal symptoms see Chapter 9; for more on treatment during childbirth see Chapter 12.
3   For more on this see P. Ekman (2003).
4   For more on pulse diagnosis see T. Kaptchuk (2000).

Chapter 9

1   Asthma UK (2004).
2   T. Dodd, *The Prevalence of Back Pain in Great Britain in 1996: A report on research for the Department of Health using the ONS omnibus survey*, The Stationery Office (1997).
3   Taken from A. Hicks (2001).

4   E.Willett,'Headaches', *Regina Leader Post and Red Deer Advocate* (2001).

5   P. Primatesta, M. Brookes, N.R. Poulter, 'Improved Hypertension Management and Control: results from the health survey for England', *Hypertension*, 38 (1998), pp. 827–32.

6   K.M. Flegal, M.D. Carroll, C.L. Ogden, C.L. Johanson, 'Prevalence and Trends in Obesity among US Adults, 1999–2001', *Journal of the American Medical Association* (2002).

7   *Storing up Problems:The medical case for a slimmer nation*, Joint Report from the Royal College of Physicians and the Royal College of Paediatrics and Child Health, RCP Publications (2004).

Chapter 11

1   For more on treating children see J. Scott (1999).

Chapter 12

1   For more on acupuncture in pregnancy and childbirth see Z.West (2001).

2   D. Habek, J. Cerkez Habek, M. Jaagust, *Acupuncture Conversion of Fetal Breech Presentation, Fetal Diagnosis and Therapy* (2003), Ch. 18, pp. 418–21.

3   *Acupuncture Electrotherapy Research*,Vol. 23(1) (1998), pp. 19–26.

4   Interestingly it is legal for anyone to give any treatment to a human – as long as the patient gives her or his permission – but only a vet can treat an animal.

Chapter 13

1   For example, acupuncture colleges like my own usually have a clinic attached. These will usually have special clinics where third-year students treat patients under the supervision of a qualified practitioner.

Bibliography

Birch, S.J., Felt, R.L., *Understanding Acupuncture*, Edinburgh: Churchill Livingstone, 1999.

Black, N., Boswell, D., Alastair, G., Murphy, S., Popay, J., *Health and Disease, A Reader*, Milton Keynes: Open University Press, 1990.

Bridges, L., *Face Reading in Chinese Medicine*, Edinburgh: Churchill Livingstone, 2004.

Ekman, P., *Emotions Revealed*, New York: Times Books, 2003.

Frantzis, B.K., *Opening the Energy Gates of Your Body*, Berkeley, California: North Atlantic Books, 2006.

Goleman, D., *Emotional Intelligence*, London: Bloomsbury, 1996.

Hicks, A., *88 Chinese Medicine Secrets*, 'How to' Books, 2010.

Hicks, A., Hicks, J., *Healing Your Emotions*, London: Thorsons, 1999.

Hicks, J., *The Principles of Chinese Herbal Medicine*, London: Thorsons, 1997.

Hicks, S., *Acupuncture Point Names*, privately published, 1999.

Hoizey, D., Hoizey, M.J., *A History of Chinese Medicine*, Edinburgh: Edinburgh University Press, 1993.

Kaptchuk, T., *The Web That Has No Weaver*, Chicago: Contemporary Publishing Group, 2000.

Larre, C., Rochat de Valle, E., *The Secret Treatise of the Spiritual Orchid*, Cambridge: Monkey Press, 1992.

Lewith, G.T., *Acupuncture, Its Place in Western Medical Science*, Edinburgh: Churchill Livingstone 1999.

Lu, H., *The Yellow Emperor's Book of Acupuncture*, Vancouver: Academy of Oriental Heritage, 1973.

Moody, R.A., *Life after Life*, London: Rider, 2001.

Scott, J., *Acupuncture in the Treatment of Children*, Seattle, Washington: Eastland Press, 1999.

West, Z., *Acupuncture in Pregnancy and Childbirth*, Edinburgh: Churchill Livingstone, 2001.

Zhang, Y.H., Rose, K., *Who Can Ride the Dragon?*, Brookline, Mass.: Paradigm Publications, 2000.

Useful Addresses

If you wish to find out more about acupuncture you can contact the professional bodies and societies listed below.

UNITED KINGDOM

British Acupuncture Council
63 Jeddo Road
London W12 9HQ
Tel: 020 8735 0400
Fax: 020 8735 0404
Email:
info@acupuncture.org.uk
www.acupuncture.org.uk

If you wish to find out more information from the author you can contact her at:
The College of Integrated Chinese Medicine
19 Castle Street
Reading
Berkshire RG1 7SB
Tel: 01189 508880
Email: admin@cicm.org.uk
www.cicm.org.uk

EUROPE

This is the pan-European organisation for all European acupuncture associations:

PEFOTS
Geldersekade 87A
1011 EK Amsterdam
Netherlands
Tel/Fax: +31 (0)20 689 2468
Email: info@pefots.com
www.pefots.com

AUSTRALIA

Australian Traditional Medicine Society
PO Box 1027
Meadowbank
New South Wales 2114
Tel: 02 9809 6800
Fax: 02 9809 7570
Email: info@atms.com.au
www.atms.com.au

Acupuncture Association of Victoria
124 Doncaster Road
Balwyn North
Victoria 3140
Tel: 05 0051 1777

Australian Acupuncture and
Chinese Medicine Association
Ltd
PO Box 1635
Corparoo DC
Queensland 4151
Tel: 0061 7 3324 2599
Fax: 0061 7 3394 2399
Email:
aacma@acupuncture.org.au
www.acupuncture.org.au

AUSTRIA

Österreichische Gesellschaft
für Akupunktur (ÖGA)
Kaiserin Elisabeth Spital
Huglgasse 1–3
A-1150 Wien
Tel: +43 1 98104 7001
Fax: +43 1 98104 5759
Email: manfred.ichart@
wienkav.at
www.akupunktur.at

Austrian Association of
Acupuncture and
Auriculotherapy
Schlosshoferstrasse 49
A1210 Vienna

BELGIUM

Ministerie van Sociale Zaken
Volksgezondheid en
Leefmilieu

Dept. van Volksgezondheid en
Leefmilieu
Pachecolaan 19, bus 5
Esplanadegeblouw
1010 Bruxelles
Tel: 02 509 8373

CANADA

General information on
acupuncture regulation etc. in
Canada:
http://www.medicinechinese.
com

The Acupuncture Foundation
of Canada Institute
2131 Laurence Avenue East
Suite 204
Scarborough
Ontario MIR SG4

Chinese Medicine and
Acupuncture Association of
Canada
www.cmaac.ca

Acupuncture Canada
www.acupuncture.ca

Ordre D'Acupunctureus Du
Quebec
1001 Boulevard
D'Masonneauve
Bureau 403
Montreal

Quebec H2L 4P9
Tel: 001 514 523 2882
Fax: 001 514 523 9669
Email:
info@ordredesacupuncteurs.qc
.ca

DENMARK

Dansk Selskab for Akupunktur
Gammel Kongevej 80
1850 Frederiksberg C
Tel: 0045 31 212112

ICMART
Gammel Kongevej 80
1850 Frederiksberg C

FINLAND

The National Research and
Development Centre for
Welfare and Health
Siltasaarenkatu 18
00531 Helsinki
Tel: 00358 900 531

FRANCE

Association Française
D'Acupuncture
9, rue del l'Église
75015 Paris Cedex 15
Tel: 01 42 52 59 07
www.acupuncture-france.com

Association de Formation
Medicale Continue et de
Recherche pour le Diplome
d'Acupuncture de l'Ouest
25 Rue Maurice Daniel
44230 St-Sebastien-sur-Loire

Societé d'Acupuncture
d'Aquitaine
www.acupuncture-aquitaine.org

GERMANY

Deutsche Ärztegesellschaft für
Akupunktur (DÄGfA)
Würmtalstrasse 54
81375 München
Tel: +49 (0)89 7 10 05 11
Fax: +49 (0)89 7 10 05 25

German Research Institute of
Chinese Medicine
Silberbachstrasse 10
79100 Freiburg im Breisgau

Deutsche Gesellschaft für
Akupunktur und Neuraltherapie
(DGfAN)
(German Society for
Acupuncture and
Neuraltherapy)
Markt 20
D-07356 Bad Lobenstein,
Germany
Tel: +49 (0)3 66 51 5 50 75
Fax: +49 (0)3 66 51 5 50 74

Arbeitsgemeinschaft fuer klassische Akupunktur und Traditionelle Chinesische Medizin e.v
Wisbacher Straße 1
83435 Bad Richenhall
D 52064 Aachen
Tel: 08651 690 919
Fax: 08651 710 694

HUNGARY

Magyar Orvosi Kamara
1063 Budapest
Szinyei Merse Pal u.4
Tel: 00361 269 4391

IRELAND

Acupuncture Foundation
Professional Association
Unit 8, Eaton House
Main Street
Rathcoole
Co. Dublin
Tel: 01 412 4917
www.acupro.ie

NETHERLANDS

NTAV
Schiedamseweg 92a
3025AG Rotterdam
Tel: +31 476 3848

Dutch Acupuncture
Association
PO Box 2198
8800 CD Amersfoort

Netherlands
Tel: +31 33 461 6141

NEW ZEALAND

New Zealand Register of Acupuncture
30 Queen's Drive,
Kilbirnie
Wellington
Tel: 0800 228 786
Email: info@acupuncture.org.nz

NORWAY

Norsk Forening for Klassik Akupunktur
Kongensg. 12
0153 Oslo
Tel: +47 22 41 78 88
Email: info@acupunktur.no
www.akupunktur.no

POLAND

Polskie Towarzystwo Akupunktury
St. Rzgowska 281/289
93–338 Lodz
Tel: +49 271 13 98
Email: lucas@akupunktura.org
www.akupunktura.org

PORTUGAL

Associação Portuguesa de Acupunctura
Rua Eca de Queiros
Nº 16B, 1º Andor

Lisboa 1050-096
Tel: +351 963 620 584
Fax: +351 213 152 269
Email: apa-da@mail.telepac.pt
www.apa-da.pt

SOUTH AFRICA
Chiropractic Homeopathic
and Allied Health Services
PO Box 17005
Groenkloof
The International Institute of
Chinese Medicine &
Acupuncture
PO Box 2246
19 Av. Disandt-Fresnaye
Cape Town 8000
Tel: 27 21 434 1654

SPAIN
Practitioners Register
Fundacion Europa de
Medicina Tradicional China
Av. de Madrid, 168–170,
Entlo A
Barcelona 08028
Tel: +34 902 16 09 42
Fax: +34 933 39 52 66

Email: mtc@mtc.com and
pr@mtc.es
www.mtc.es

USA
Council of Colleges of
Acupuncture and Oriental
Medicine
600 Wyndhurst Avenue,
Suite 112
Baltimore, MD 21210

National Acupuncture and
Oriental Medicine Alliance
1833 North 105th Street
Seattle, WA 98133

National Commission for the
Certification of Acupuncturists
(NCCAOM)
76 South Laura Street
Suite 1290
Jacksonville, FL 32202
Tel: 001 904 598 1005
Fax: 001 904 598 5001
Email: info@nccaom.org
www.nccaom.org

Index

Note: page numbers in **bold** refer to diagrams.

ACUPRESSURE

How to cure common ailments the natural way

Michael Reed Gach, PhD

In *Acupressure*, bestselling author and acupressure expert Michael Reed Gach explains this ancient healing art which uses the fingers to press key points on the surface of the skin and stimulate the body's natural self-curative abilities.

The technique is both safe and easy to learn, with no drug-induced side effects, and offers you the potential to improve your health and increase your vitality.

It includes:

- Simple techniques to relieve problems such as headaches,arthritis, colds, fatigue, insomnia, backache and depression.

- Pressure-point maps and exercises to relieve pain and restore function.

- A 5-minute acupressure routine to maintain health and relieve stress

- A way to complement conventional medical care and take a vital role in becoming well and staying well.

978-0-7499-2534-5

THE REFLEXOLOGY HANDBOOK

A complete guide

Laura Norman and Thomas Cowan

The Reflexology Handbook explains simply, and with clear drawings and diagrams, how you can use this easily accessible holistic technique to relive a wide range of physical problems.

Top reflexologist Laura Norman shows how everyone can use foot reflexology to relive common conditions such as headaches, respiratory ailments, osteoporosis, insomnia, gallstones, sports injuries, weight problems and high blood pressure. She also includes:

- Advice on how reflexology can reduce stress, revitalise energy and strengthen relationships in families and couples

- Clear descriptions of the reflex points and the basic reflexology techniques

- Specific chapters for different situation, conditions and people

- A chart of common ailments and the reflexology techniques to relieve them

'Enjoyable and easy to read . . . I would recommend it to any reflexologist' Nicola M Hall, The British Reflexology Association

978-0-7499-2378-0